ANTI INFLAMMATORY DIET COOKBOOK

The Book of Easy, Delicious and Tasty Recipes for Beginners, for Establishing New Eating Habits Based on Good Meals and Delicious Recipes

RIHANNA SMITH

TABLE OF CONTENCT

Introduction

What is Inflammation?

In the simplest terms, Inflammation is the process of how the body's immune system reacts whenever it detects the presence of a foreign entity inside the body or any form of injury. During an inflammatory response, White Blood Cells alongside a number of different substances tries to protect the body from further damage that might result from the contamination.

However, things change when this very action takes a turn for the worst.

Whenever you are dealing with something such as Arthritis, which is also related to chronic inflammation, the defense mechanism of the body seems to malfunction and trigger an inflammatory response even though there are no contamination.

Diseases that tend to do these are largely known as "Auto Immune" diseases and instead of protecting the body, the body's own auto-immune system starts to harm itself and damage the tissues

That being said, let's have a look at some of the main reasons of Inflammation.

What causes inflammation?

Various factors come into play when considering the reasons as to "What" causes inflammation in a human being. More often than not, a vast majority of the reasons tend to directly linked to poor Lifestyle choices, however, it should be noted that aging is a big factor here as well.

Some of the most crucial causes to know about include:

Aging

The natural process of aging contributes to Inflammation as well. As we age, few of our cells tend to regenerate and most of them start to die, leaving behind waste materials that tend to trigger inflammation.

Obesity and Inactivity

Excessive inactivity can and will often lead to obesity, which itself is a major cause of inflammation.

Adipose tissue, the layer of fat that is found right under our skin is actually responsible for much more than just keeping it warm.

It is a metabolically active layer that causes the body to change the body chemistry and is also affected by the body's other systems.

The fat layer contains a large number of white blood cells and greater number of fat (obviously).

However, the cell count is actually linked together. Meaning, the more fat there are, the greater number of white cells will be present.

These cells often tend to release pro-inflammatory substances that gradually contribute to the rise of inflammatory effects.

Diet

If we make a comparison, we would soon see that most of the causes of Inflammation are related to diet, so we are keeping this on the top of the list.

Harmful substances such as refined fats, animal products and refined carbohydrates tend to do a lot of damage in the long run.

It should be noted though that carbohydrates don't directly contribute to inflammation, but refined foods with higher concentration and fats are found to be naturally dense with inflammation causing substance that affect that gut and increases inflammation.

The types of fat that are consumed by an individual also plays a greater role here. Back in the early days when everything was simple, people used to stay on a diet that was very well balanced on both Omega 3 and Omega 6 fats. However, modern diets tend to have a very high concentration of Omega -6 fat as oppose to the Omega 3 fat, this increase the possibility of suffering from inflammation by 10-20%!

It's very important for the body to have a good supply of Omega-3 fatty acids because the Omega 6 and Omega 3, both compete for the same COX enzymes, which are needed to build large fatty molecules.

COX-2 enzyme in particular are essential for making inflammatory prostaglandins.

Too much of Omega-6 fatty acids will result in the domination of this enzyme and the body won't be able to utilize these enzymes anymore in conjunction with Omega-3 fats to reduce inflammation.

Nowadays fats are even chemically modified and this plays a greater role to inflammation as well. They are made to be more inexpensive, which results in the production of highly inflammatory products.

Stress

Cortisol is a hormone that is produced by adrenal glands and is used to manage the body's response to stress.

It helps to stimulate burst of energy and suppresses the action of pro-inflammatory substance.

This also helps to reduce stress by counter acting the effects of pro-inflammatory eicosanoids. However, if you stress too much, the amount of cortisol might increase to a dramatic level that will cause your immune cells to lose the sensitivity to this hormone and trigger inflammation.

Smoking

Exposure to various toxins such as cigarette smoke plays a great role in Inflammation. Either second hand or firsthand, inhaled tobacco tend to tends to extensively cripple the body's capacity to fight diseases by suppressing the production of white blood cells.

So, it's best to avoid smoking as much as possible.

Main Principles of the Anti-Inflammatory Diet

The anti-inflammatory diet is not merely a meal plan to maintain within a limited duration; additionally, it is not solely weight loss program as well.

Nevertheless, you can indeed lose weight by practicing it. Instead, the diet is a systematic way of choosing the right foods and preparing anti-inflammatory meals.

It derives its food selection and cooking processes on the scientific and medical knowledge of how your food intakes can help your body to attain and maintain optimum wellness. This natural dieting greatly influences the beneficial goals of inflammation.

The regimen provides you with a steady supply of energy, mainly sourced from the sufficient macronutrient consumptions. These intakes include dietary fibers and essential fatty acids. You will also have your ample share of vitamins and minerals from the micronutrient intakes.

Likewise, you can benefit more with the diet's protective phytonutrients. These are healthy and nourishing substances commonly derived from plants such as lycopene, lutein, and carotene.

People suffering from inflammatory diseases can reduce their inflammation and its side effects. They only need to radically change their diets. They can enhance the effect of taking prescribed medications with a proper nutrition program (anti-inflammatory diet).

Logically, if you intend to reduce inflammation, then consume less of the inflammatory foods. Instead, eat more and more of the anti-inflammatory foods.

Your regimen must provide for a healthy balance of macronutrients—fats, proteins, and carbohydrates—at each meal. Ensure also to meet your body's daily requirements for fibers, water, vitamins, and minerals.

Base your anti-inflammatory diet on nutrient-rich and whole foods containing antioxidants. These substances ably help to protect your cells from the destructive effects of oxidation.

In essence, antioxidants function by reducing the levels of free radicals. These are incredibly reactive compounds, which damage fats and proteins.

Free radicals also accelerate the progression of cardiovascular diseases, rheumatoid arthritis, cancer, radiation sickness, atherosclerosis, age-related illnesses, and many other health issues. Hence, avoid processed products, which are often dense with free radicals.

Generally, the natural design and function of the highly reactive molecules of free radicals are to assist metabolism. This biological process involves breaking down food compounds into smaller particles and disposing the absorbed nutrients into the blood to create energy for your body.

However, when you are unable to reduce or purge any intense reactions of these harmful free radicals, they can ultimately lead to inflammatory issues. You can only hold them in check through ingesting prescribed foods from the regimen.

Various Versions & Variations Of The Dietary Discipline: Replacement Regimens

The anti-inflammatory diet is a natural and nutritional regimen. As such, it encompasses most dietary plans.

The diet is relative to a wide range of recommended traditional and modern nutritional regimen. Its breadths and depths reflect the recommended food compositions.

The food elements include lots of fruits and vegetables, plant-based proteins (i.e., nuts and legumes), and fresh, organically grown herbs and spices. Whole grains and fatty fish are also among the regular staples.

If you were to account the macronutrient values, then the regimen inherently has limited calories (energy content of food), proteins, and saturated fats (solid fats). However, it is significantly rich in fibers or plant carbohydrates and trans-unsaturated fats (essential fatty acids).

Incidentally, these typical foods also form part of the core of food elements of several dietary disciplines. Three of these popular diets are the Mediterranean Diet, various types of Low-Carbohydrate Diets, and Vegan/Vegetarian Diets. Many nutritionists and dieticians consider these regimens as anti-inflammatory diets in nature.

Mediterranean Meals: The conception of the Mediterranean Diet was an inspiration of the time-honored dietary habits of people living within the Mediterranean region. The main feature of the diet is the high consumptions of olive oil, unrefined grains, legumes, fruits, and vegetables.

The regimen also includes moderate-to-high intakes of seafood and dairy products (often, yogurt and cheese). However, it restricts consuming non-fish and red meats. Its distinctive aspect emphasizes social celebrations of food with regulated intakes of wine.

Generally, it is a beneficial dietary plan rich in dietary fibers and monounsaturated fats while low in saturated fats. The Mediterranean Diet demonstrates to reduce inflammatory indicators like IL-6 and CRP.

Olive oil is the primary component of the diet that promotes good health. Studies insist that the regular consumptions of olive oil can lower mortality rates, neurodegeneration, and cardiovascular diseases. Additional studies also show that olive oil reduces the risks of cancer and several other chronic diseases.

Common Carb-Restricted Regimens: As its term implies, the dietary program emphasizes carbohydrate restriction. People often apply this typical regimen for the treatment or prevention of some chronic diseases.

These recurring health issues include high blood pressure and cardiovascular disease, gut fermentation and metabolic syndromes, and diabetes. It also reduces inflammation, especially for people who are obese.

The working principle of this diet entails limiting or replacing foods high in carbohydrates with foods that are rich in fats but moderate in proteins, as well as other foods low in carbs. The replaced food items are usually those easily digestible foods (i.e., pasta, bread, sugar, etc.), which have high glycemic indices (carb ratings that measure how quickly they raise blood sugar levels).

On one hand, these diets highly suggest consuming fatty foods with adequate protein contents. These food sources generally come from dairy, livestock, and poultry produce; nuts and seeds; and, seafood, particularly shellfish.

On the other hand, these diets recommended low-carb foods are those dark, green, and leafy vegetables. Low-carb diets also advise intakes of specific fruits, most preferably, berries.

The tolerable amounts of carb intakes vary with each specific low-carb regimen. Generally, a low-carb diet applies to meal plans that limit carb consumptions to less than 20% of one's recommended daily calorie intake.

For a steady and healthy dietary regimen, males require about 2,500 calories per day for healthy weight maintenance. Females need only to consume 2,000 calories each day. However, these figures may vary depending on age, body composition, and intensity levels of daily physical activities.

Similarly, low-carb diets may also refer to regimens that limit carb intakes to not more than the maximum recommended values. They use a rule of thumb for carb restrictions between 5% and 30% of your daily calorie intake.

The Ketogenic Diet is the chief proponent of this severe carb restriction regimen. The diet follows a regulated food consumption of 70% to 80% of calories from fats, 15% to 25% of calories from proteins, and 5% to 10% of calories from carbohydrates.

These caloric ratios fulfill the intents of inducing the body to enter into a state of ketosis. Ketosis is the occurrence of an excessive accumulation of ketones or fatty tissues in the bloodstream that the body cells use to burn for energy instead of carbohydrates.

The Atkins Diet also has a similar induction stage as the Ketogenic Diet. The only difference between these low-carb diets is the prescribed amounts of protein consumptions. The Atkins Diet proffers unlimited protein intakes along its 4-stage dietary plan.

The Paleo Diet is also a relatively low-carb regimen. It has a carb intake rating of 20% to 40% of calories from carbs.

The regimen distinctively summons the analogy of the eating patterns of our ancient ancestors who were initially hunter-gatherers. Thus, the diet mainly focuses on plant and animal foods low in carbs. Studies show that wild and organically grown plants contain fewer carbs and abundant in fiber compared to modern plant crops.

Vegan | Vegetarian Versions: Vegan and Vegetarian Diets carry the same wellness intent: to reduce inflammation. Engaging with the anti-inflammatory diet is like indulging with vegan protein sources or fatty fish instead of meat.

The principal staples of both Vegan and Vegetarian Diets are plant-based foods rich in vitamin K. These are mostly dark, green, and leafy veggies like broccoli, kale, and spinach. These leafy greens have long been heralded to help restrain inflammation.

Fresh fruits (i.e., blackberries, raspberries, etc.) are also essential food items of these plant-based regimens. The pigment that produces the specific colors for these fruits is a vital element in battling inflammation.

These versions and variations of the diet have already gained a foothold and a broader acceptance in today's society. Practitioners use them either as strategies to maintain good health or as medical nutrition therapies to manage their health issues. Nonetheless, most people commit themselves actively to these diets to seek protection against inflammatory conditions.

Summing it up, numerous studies have validated the countless health benefits of each of these regimens. For one, experts confirmed that vegetarians had increased levels of plasma amino acid (general health indicators associated with lower risks of heart disease and inflammation). In contrast, a recent study affirmed that consuming animal products increased the chances of acquiring chronic inflammation.

Gaining & Growing On Bountiful Benefits

Naturopaths, dietitians, nutritionists, and physicians are always inclined to prescribe the anti-inflammatory regimen. In all likelihood, they will endorse it as a complementary therapy for several health conditions aggravated by chronic inflammation.

Since it is a widely regarded healthy diet, it helps to lessen your chances of acquiring other health problems. That is, even if the regimen does not help with your current conditions.

The principal benefit of an anti-inflammatory diet is the reduction of inflammatory indicators in the blood. Foremost, it enhances blood sugar, triglyceride, and cholesterol levels.

The dietary regimen also boosts energy while improving your overall health and moods. In conclusion, strictly following an anti-inflammatory regimen and lifestyle, together with regular physical exercise and adequate sleep, can drastically reduce your risks of incurring many diseases, to wit:

- Active Hepatitis
- Alzheimer's disease
- Asthma
- Cancer, particularly Colorectal Cancer
- Chronic Sinusitis | Ulcerative Colitis
- Colitis
- Crohn's Disease
- Diabetes
- Eosinophilic Esophagitis
- Hashimoto's Disease
- Heart Diseases
- Inflammatory Bowel Syndromes (IBS)
- Lupus
- Metabolic Syndrome
- Obesity

- Peptic Ulcer
- Periodontitis
- Psoriasis
- Rheumatoid Arthritis
- Tuberculosis

The Anti-Inflammatory Diet Foods to Eat and Avoid

The anti-inflammatory diet can be restricted for specific types of foods. This is to ensure that you don't introduce things that might trigger inflammatory responses to your body. Although there are some types of foods that you should avoid with this particular diet, there is still a plethora of food groups that you are allowed to enjoy while following this diet.

Food groups	Anti-inflammation all-stars	Foods to avoid
Beans and legumes	Black-eyed peas, red beans, pinto beans, lentils, chickpeas, and black beans	NA
Fruits	Blueberries, blackberries, raspberries, strawberries, dark red grapes, cherries, coconut, avocado, and citrus fruits	NA
Allium vegetables	Onion, garlic, chives, shallots, leeks, green onions	NA
Vegetables	Cauliflower, broccoli, and cabbage. Also, dark leafy greens like mustard greens, collard greens, kale, lettuce, and spinach. Mushrooms, squash	NA
Nightshade vegetables	Tomatoes, bell peppers, eggplants, and potatoes	There is no scientific evidence that shows the nightshade group of vegetables have

		inflammatory properties. In fact, they are a nutritional powerhouse. Thus, if an individual is sensitive to nightshade food, then it is prudent to remove it from your diet.
Herbs and spices	Thyme, rosemary, cinnamon, basil, garlic, ginger, turmeric, chili peppers, paprika,	NA
Animal and fish products	Oily fish like herring, salmon, tuna, mackerel, and sardines. Lean meat	Avoid processed meats like sausages as they contain nitrites – a form of preservative that does little good to the body. Red meat like burgers and steaks
Recommended fats	Fats from coconut, avocado, olive oils. Fats from nuts like almonds, pine nuts, pistachios, and walnuts. Cocoa and chocolates	Fats found in fried foods; vegetable oil and soybean oil, margarine, shortening, and lard. Fats found in whole milk, butter—consider using low-fat dairy. Food laden with trans-fat such as processed foods should be avoided completely.
Recommended drinks	Green tea Red wine in moderation	Sugary drinks Excessive alcohol
Carbohydrates	Whole grains like unrefined grains, whole wheat bread, brown rice, oatmeal.	Refined carbs like white bread and pastries. French fries Artificial sugar should also be avoided.

The Science Behind the Anti-Inflammatory Diet

When your body needs to respond to an injury, it tends to mobilize an army of specialized cells to fend of the invading organism and toxins.

These cells prepare pathways for fighter cells to attack and completely engulf the attackers.

Once that has happened, another group of cells tend to signal to the body and let it know the fighter cells have accomplished their task and the body is allowed to stop the production of preparatory and fighter cells.

These results a sort of cleanup that clears up the leftover fighter cells from the battlefield and repairs any damage.

Simply put, there are two steps to this response:

Pro-Inflammatory

Anti-Inflammatory

Each cell involved in the pro stage builds on the work of the previous cells and helps to make the immune reaction stronger for any upcoming attack.

During the pro period, symptoms such as redness, swelling, itching are common.

The anti-inflammatory is the reverse of pro-inflammatory and it works to lower the effects of inflammation.

A variety of substances used to block inflammation are made from essential fatty acids, which the body isn't able to produce on its own.

These acids must be obtained through supplements or foods.

Two essential ones are Omega-3 and Omega-6.

Omega-6 tends to increase inflammation while Omega-3 helps to reduce it.

It should be noted that what I wrote above is a simplified version of the whole mechanism and there is a lot more to it.

There are various substances that play a deeper role in the whole infrastructure that allows the body to control its inflammatory mechanism.

Some of the crucial ones are:

Histamine: White blood cells near an injury tend to release a substance known as histamine. They increase the permeability of blood vessels around the wound that signals fighter cells and other substances to regulate an immune response and come to the sight of injury. Histamine also causes redness and swelling around the affected region and causes runny nose, rash, itchy eyes.

Cytokines: These are proteins that are activated by pro-inflammatory eicosanoids to signal fighter cells to gather at the injury site. They are responsible for diverting energy from the body to catalyst the healing process. Release of these substances tend to cause tiredness and decrease appetite.

C-Reactive Protein: Cytokines alongside other pro-inflammatory eicosanoids are closely involved in the activation of a substance known as C-Reactive Protein. This particular organic compound produced by the liver responds to messages that are sent out by white blood cells. The C-Reactive proteins tend to bind the site of injury and act as a sort of surveillance unit that helps to identify the invading bodies.

Leukocytes: Several types of leukocytes (also known as white blood cells) are critical to the process of neutralizing invading substances. Neutrophils, for example, are small, agile and are able to first arrive at the scene of the crime to ingest small microbes. However, large substances such as macrophages as required to tackle a large number of microbes.

There are a few more, but the gist still remains the same. When your body starts to suffer from an uncontrolled inflammation attack, the action of these and similar substances tend to get out of control, which results in extremely uncomfortable situations.

Anti-Inflammatory Foods

An inflammatory response is caused by the activation of white blood cells in response to foreign entities in the body.

Whenever a molecule enters our bloodstream, our white blood cells immediately start to recognize that molecule as either belonging to the body or alien. If the molecule is foreign, it is tagged and removed to prevent it from causing any harm. The white blood cells also cause a series of processes, which are intended to minimize damage and contain pathogens.

For example, the chemicals released by the white blood cells often cause fluid to flow into the affected areas, therefore causing swelling. Likewise, redness often occurs due to increased blood flow (this helps white blood cells move to the appropriate place).

It is important to note that inflammation doesn't just affect the skin and joints, but it can also affect the internal organs. As you might expect, inflammation of the internal organs can cause serious health problems. Inflammation of the heart, for example, is called myocarditis and is associated with shortness of breath. Conversely, inflammation of the kidneys is also associated with high blood pressure and even outright kidney failure.

In some circumstances the inflammatory response arises due to a false positive, such as particular allergens, arthritis or an excessive intake of certain foods.

Inflammation is associated with redness, swollen warm joints, joint pain or stiffness and overall lack of malleability in the joints.

Inflammation has also been connected with a general reduction in well-being due to a myriad of flu-like symptoms such as pain, fatigue, headaches, fever and loss of appetite.

Therefore, if you find yourself suffering from any of these inflammatory symptoms then it can be useful to incorporate anti-inflammatory foods into your diet.

Current understanding is that there are dozens of potential sources of inflammation and just as many molecules that can help mediate both the causes and symptoms.

In particular, food scientists often record the presence of two proteins in the bloodstream (C-reactive protein & interluekin-6) as accurate indicators of the level of inflammation people suffer.

These two proteins are known to be controlled by omega-3 fatty acids, which are also known to have several other benefits (such as improving cognition).

Omega-3 fatty acids are present in several types of fish, including but not limited to

Salmon

Sardines

Tuna

Anchovies

Additionally, numerous nuts have omega-3, especially walnuts and almonds.

Inflammation is also thought to be reduced by a stronger and more efficient immune system. The exact mechanism by which a better immune system alleviates inflammatory response is not known, although there are a few hypotheses.

Namely, it is thought, that a more efficient immune system may manage problems faster, resulting in less time spent in an inflammatory response. Alternatively, a more productive immune system might produce fewer 'false positives' and react less severely to molecules, which are not genuinely harmful.

Regardless of the method, there is therefore reason to believe in a link between molecules that support the immune system (such as anti-oxidants) and lower levels of inflammation. The foods highest in anti-oxidants tend to be herbs & spices, although there are exceptions.

In particular the following foods are known to be especially potent;

Cloves

Ginger

Rosemary

Turmeric

Cinnamon

Allspice

Marjoram

Sage

Thyme

Italian Spice

Although you can supplement your meals with herbs and spices, their effect will be limited due to the small amount actually consumed. Therefore, it is also important to incorporate other foods, which are less powerful but can be eaten in greater quantities.

Many fruits & vegetables contain also contain high amounts of antioxidants and they can also feasibly be eaten in more meaningful quantities. Strong antioxidant choices include blueberries, blackberries, cherries, strawberries, spinach, kale & broccoli.

Additionally, foods high in monounsaturated fat should also be included in an anti-inflammatory diet. The exact reason why monounsaturated fat seems to have an anti-inflammatory effect is not known, although it has been suggested to be partially due to the presence of antioxidants and partially due to how monounsaturated fat promotes the absorption of vitamins & minerals (promoting overall bodily health).

Foods high in monosatured fat include nuts, seeds, olives, avocados and some types of vegetable oils. In particular, walnuts & almonds should make particularly prominent choices due to the fact that they also contain omega-3 and omega-6 fatty acids, which as previously mentioned, also have anti-inflammatory properties.

Other anti-inflammatory foods include most types of beans (such as kidney beans or butter beans). Beans are low in the glycaemic index, which categorizes foods by how quickly the carbohydrates within them are absorbed.

It is widely believed that inflammation may be partially due to excessive sugar and carbohydrate intake, foods with low glycaemic index values arguably have anti-inflammatory properties too.

Likewise, beans are high in fibre, which may promote overall gastrointestinal health and reduce intestinal inflammation. Fibre also lowers levels of the previously before-mentioned C-reactive protein (or CRP for short).

As a general rule of thumb, colorful fruits and vegetables are typically associated with both high levels of anti-oxidants as well as high levels of fiber, making them fantastic at lowering inflammation.

Moreover, several types of red wine can also be considered to be anti-inflammatory. Red wine, especially red wine originating from the Mediterranean and France, has been noted for its high levels of anti-oxidants.4

However, red wine also contains a molecule called Resveratrol, which is under research for its anti-inflammatory properties. With this being said, keeping alcohol intake within a reasonable level is obviously important for overall health.

Additionally, leafy greens (such as spinach, kale, collard greens & Swiss chard) are rich in multiple types of molecules that reduce inflammation.

Finally, consider adding tea (such as matcha tea & tulsi tea), blueberries, fermented foods, shiitake mushrooms & garlic.

To add to all of this, you might want to consider cutting some foods from your diet. Many of the usual unhealthy foods are suspected to increase inflammatory symptoms, such as processed foods, foods high in unhealthy fats and sodium.

Nonetheless, there are also some offenders you might not expect. The so-called nightshade branch of foods (which includes eggplant, tomatoes, peppers &) has been accused of exacerbating inflammation and arthritis. However, actual scientific support for this claim is rather sketchy.

To conclude, an anti-inflammatory diet would consist of a diet centered on the following foods;

Herbs & Spices

Fish

Nuts, Seeds, Avocado & Vegetable Oil

Fruit & Vegetables

Beans

Red Wine

Leafy Greens

The remainder of this eBook will provide you with numerous recipes high in these anti-inflammatory foods.

Breakfast Recipes

1. Morning Bowl

Preparation Time: 5 minutes

Cooking Time: 0

Servings: 1

Ingredients: 1 cup coconut milk

1 teaspoon raw honey

1 teaspoon walnuts; chopped.

1 teaspoon pistachios; chopped.

1 teaspoon almonds; chopped.

1 teaspoon pine nuts; raw

1 teaspoon pepitas; raw

2 teaspoons raspberries

1 teaspoon pecans; chopped.

1 teaspoon sunflower seeds; raw

Directions:

In a bowl, mix milk with honey and stir.

Add pecans, walnuts, almonds, pistachios, sunflower seeds, pine nuts and pepitas

Stir, top with raspberries and serve

Nutrition: Calories: 100 Cal Fat: 2 g

Fiber: 4 g Carbs: 5 g Protein: 6 g

2. Breakfast Stir Fry

Preparation Time: 20 Minutes

Cooking Time: 20 Minutes

Servings: 2

Ingredients:

1/2 pounds beef meat; minced

1 tablespoon tamari sauce

2 bell peppers; chopped.

2 teaspoons red chili flakes

1 teaspoon chili powder

1 tablespoon coconut oil

Salt and black pepper to the taste.

For the bok choy:

6 bunches bok choy; trimmed and chopped.

1 teaspoon ginger; grated

1-tablespoon coconut oil

Salt to the taste.

For the eggs:

2 eggs

1 tablespoon coconut oil

Directions:

Heat up a pan with 1 tablespoon coconut oil over medium high heat; add beef and bell peppers; stir and cook for 10 minutes

Add salt, pepper, tamari sauce, chili flakes and chili powder; stir, cook for 4 minutes more and take off heat.

Heat up another pan with 1 tablespoon oil over medium heat; add bok choy; stir and cook for 3 minutes

Add salt and ginger; stir, cook for 2 minutes more and take off heat.

Heat up the third pan with 1 tablespoon oil over medium heat; crack eggs and fry them.

Divide beef and bell peppers mix into 2 bowls

Divide bok choy and top with eggs

Nutrition:

Calories: 248 Cal

Fat: 14 g

Fiber: 4 g

Carbs: 10 g

Protein: 14 g

3. Cereal Nibs

Preparation Time: 25 minutes

Cooking Time: 30 Minutes

Servings: 4

Ingredients:

4 tablespoons hemp hearts

1/2 cup chia seeds

2 tablespoons coconut oil

1 tablespoon swerve

2 tablespoons cocoa nibs

1 tablespoon vanilla extract

1 tablespoon psyllium powder

1 cup water

Directions:

In a bowl, mix chia seeds with water; stir and leave aside for 5 minutes

Add hemp hearts, vanilla extract, psyllium powder, oil and swerve and stir well with your mixer.

Add cocoa nibs, and stir until you obtain a dough.

Divide dough into 2 pieces, shape into cylinder form, place on a lined baking sheet, flatten well, cover with a parchment paper, introduce in the oven at 285 degrees F and bake for 20 minutes

Remove the parchment paper and bake for 25 minutes more

Take cylinders out of the oven, leave aside to cool down and cut into small pieces

Serve in the morning with some almond milk.

Nutrition:

Calories: 245 Cal Fat: 12 g

Fiber: 12 g Carbs: 2 g Protein: 9 g

4. Chicken Muffins

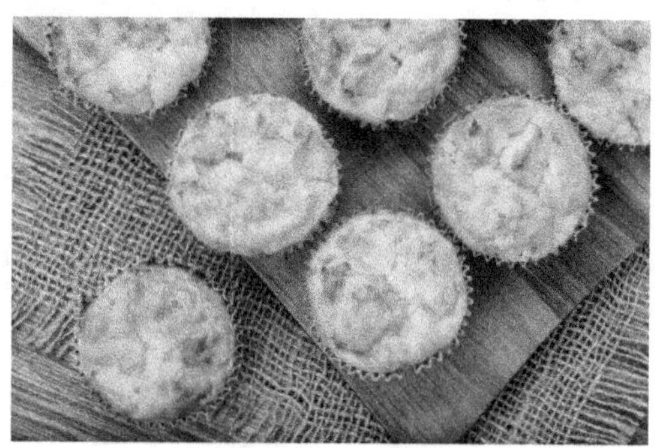

Preparation Time: 15 Minutes

Cooking Time: 55 Minutes

Servings: 3

Ingredients:

3/4-pound chicken breast; boneless

1/2 teaspoon garlic powder

2 tablespoons green onions; chopped.

3 tablespoons hot sauce mixed with 3 tablespoons melted coconut oil

6 eggs

Salt and black pepper to the taste.

Directions:

Season chicken breast with salt, pepper and garlic powder, place on a lined baking sheet and bake in the oven at 425 degrees F for 25 minutes

Transfer chicken breast to a bowl, shred with a fork and mix with half of the hot sauce and melted coconut oil.

Toss to coat and leave aside for now.

In a bowl, mix eggs with salt, pepper, green onions and the rest of the hot sauce mixed with oil and whisk very well.

Divide this mix into a muffin tray, top each with shredded chicken, introduce in the oven at 350 degrees F and bake for 30 minutes

Serve your muffins hot.

Nutrition:

Calories: 140 Cal

Fat: 8 g

Fiber: 1 g

Carbs: 2 g

Protein: 13 g

5. Egg Porridge

Preparation Time: 14 minutes

Cooking Time: 0

Servings: 2

Ingredients:

2 eggs

2 tablespoons ghee; melted

1/3 cup heavy cream

1 tablespoon stevia

A pinch of cinnamon; ground

Directions:

In a bowl, mix eggs with stevia and heavy cream and whisk well.

Heat up a pan with the ghee over medium high heat; add egg mix and cook until they are done

Transfer to 2 bowls, sprinkle cinnamon on top and serve

Nutrition:

Calories: 340 Cal

Fat: 12 g Fiber: 10;

Carbs: 3 g

6. Waffles

Preparation Time: 20 Minutes

Cooking Time: 10 Minutes

Servings: 5

Ingredients:

5 eggs; separated

4 ounces ghee; melted

3 tablespoons almond milk

1 teaspoon baking powder

4 tablespoons coconut flour

2 teaspoon vanilla

3 tablespoons stevia

Directions:

In a bowl, whisk egg white using your mixer.

In another bowl mix flour with stevia, baking powder and egg yolks and whisk well.

Add vanilla, ghee and milk and stir well again.

Add egg white and stir gently everything.

Pour some of the mix into your waffle maker and cook until it's golden.

Repeat with the rest of the batter and serve your waffles right away.

Nutrition:

Calories: 240 Cal Fat: 23 g

Fiber: 2 g Carbs: 4 g Protein: 7 g

7. Quick Burrito

Preparation Time:10 Minutes

Cooking Time: 11 Minutes

Servings: 1

Ingredients: 1/4-pound beef meat; ground

1 teaspoon sweet paprika

1 teaspoon cumin; ground

1 teaspoon onion powder

1 small red onion; julienned 3 eggs

1 teaspoon coconut oil

1 teaspoon garlic powder

1 teaspoon cilantro; chopped.

Salt and black pepper to the taste.

Directions:

Heat up a pan over medium heat; add beef and brown for a few minutes

Add salt, pepper, cumin, garlic and onion powder and paprika; stir, cook for 4 minutes more and take off heat.

In a bowl, mix eggs with salt and pepper and whisk well. Heat up a pan with the oil over medium heat; add egg, spread evenly and cook for 6 minutes Transfer your egg burrito to a plate, divide beef mix, add onion and cilantro, roll and serve

Nutrition: Calories: 280 Cal Fat: 12 g

Fiber: 4 g Carbs: 7 g Protein: 14 g

8. Poached Eggs

Preparation Time: 10 Minutes

Cooking Time 40 Minutes

Servings: 4

Ingredients: 3 tomatoes; chopped.

3 garlic cloves; minced

1 tablespoon ghee 1/4 teaspoon chili powder

1 tablespoon cilantro; chopped. 6 eggs

1 white onion; chopped.

1 red bell pepper; chopped.

1 teaspoon paprika

1 teaspoon cumin

1 Serrano pepper; chopped.

Salt and black pepper to the taste.

Directions:

Heat up a pan with the ghee over medium heat; add onion; stir and cook for 10 minutes

Add Serrano pepper and garlic; stir and cook for 1 minute

Add red bell pepper; stir and cook for 10 minutes

Add tomatoes, salt, pepper, chili powder, cumin and paprika; stir and cook for 10 minutes

Crack eggs into the pan, season them with salt and pepper, cover pan and cook for 6 minutes more

Sprinkle cilantro at the end and serve

Nutrition:

Calories: 300 Cal Fat: 12 g Fiber: 4 g

Carbs: 22 g Protein: 14 g

9. Pumpkin Pancakes

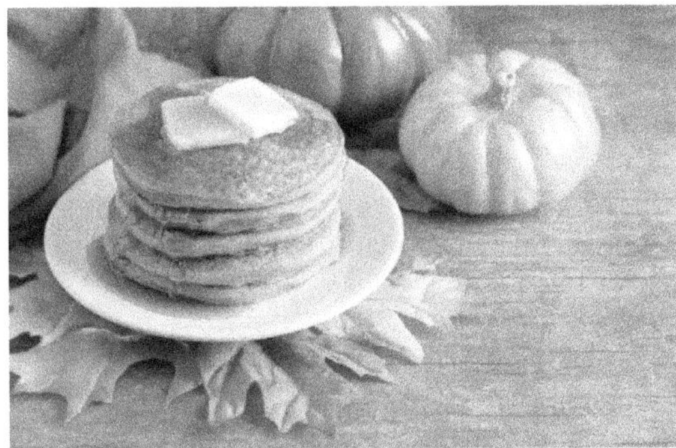

Preparation Time: 20 Minutes

Cooking Time: 5 Minutes

Servings: 6

Ingredients:

2 ounces hazelnut flour

2 ounces flax seeds; ground

1-ounce egg white protein

1 teaspoon coconut oil

1 tablespoon chai masala

1 teaspoon vanilla extract

1 teaspoon baking powder

1 cup coconut cream

1 tablespoon swerve

1/2 cup pumpkin puree

3 eggs

5 drops stevia

Directions:

In a bowl, mix flax seeds with hazelnut flour, egg white protein, baking powder and chai masala and stir.

In another bowl, mix coconut cream with vanilla extract, pumpkin puree, eggs, stevia and swerve and stir well.

Combine the 2 mixtures and stir well.

Heat up a pan with the oil over medium high heat; pour 1/6 of the batter, spread into a circle, cover, reduce heat to low, cook for 3 minutes on each side and transfer to a plate

Repeat with the rest of the batter and serve your pumpkin pancakes right away.

Nutrition:

Calories: 400 Cal

Fat: 23 g

Fiber: 4 g

Carbs: 5 g

Protein: 21 g

10. Cauliflower and Chorizo

Preparation Time: 15 Minutes

Cooking Time: 40 Minutes

Servings: 4

Ingredients:

1 cauliflower head; florets separated

4 eggs; whisked

1/2 teaspoon garlic powder

2 tablespoons green onions; chopped.

1-pound chorizo; chopped.

12 ounces canned green chilies; chopped.

1 yellow onion; chopped.

Salt and black pepper to the taste.

Directions:

Heat up a pan over medium heat; add chorizo and onion; stir and brown for a few minutes

Add green chilies; stir, cook for a few minutes and take off heat.

In your food processor mix cauliflower with some salt and pepper and blend.

Transfer this to a bowl, add eggs, salt, pepper and garlic powder and whisk everything.

Add chorizo mix as well, whisk again and transfer everything to a greased baking dish.

Bake in the oven at 375 degrees F and bake for 40 minutes

Leave casserole to cool down for a few minutes, sprinkle green onions on top, slice and serve

Nutrition:

Calories: 350 Cal Fat: 12 g Fiber: 4 g

Carbs: 6 g Protein: 20 g

11. No Cook Overnight Oats

Preparation Time: 5 Minutes

Cooking Time: 0

Servings: 1

Ingredients: 1 ½ c. low fat milk

5 whole almond pieces   1 tsp. chia seeds

2 tbsps. Oats   1 tsp. sunflower seeds

1 tbsp. Craisins

Directions:

In a jar or mason bottle with cap, mix all ingredients. Refrigerate overnight.

Enjoy for breakfast. Will keep in the fridge for up to 3 days.

Nutrition:

Calories: 271 Cal Fat:9.8 g Carbs:35.4 g

Protein:16.7 g Sugars:9 g

12. Avocado Cup with Egg

Preparation Time: 5 Minutes

Cooking Time: 25 Minutes

Servings: 4

Ingredients:

4 tsps. parmesan cheese

1 chopped stalk scallion

4 dashes pepper

4 dashes paprika

2 ripe avocados

4 medium eggs

Directions:

Preheat oven to 375 0F.

Slice avocadoes in half and discard seed.

Slice the rounded portions of the avocado, to make it level and sit well on a baking sheet.

Place avocadoes on baking sheet and crack one egg in each hole of the avocado.

Season each egg evenly with pepper, and paprika.

Pop in the oven and bake for 25 minutes or until eggs are cooked to your liking.

Serve with a sprinkle of parmesan.

Nutrition: Calories: 206 Cal

Fat:15.4 g Carbs:11.3 g Protein:8.5 g

Sugars:0.4 g

13. Mediterranean toast

Preparation Time: 10 Minutes

Cooking Time: 0

Servings: 2

Ingredients:

1 ½ tsp. reduced-fat crumbled feta

3 sliced Greek olives

¼ mashed avocado

1 slice good whole wheat bread

1 tbsp. roasted red pepper hummus

3 sliced cherry tomatoes

1 sliced hardboiled egg

Directions:

First, toast the bread and top it with ¼ mashed avocado and 1 tablespoon hummus.

Add the cherry tomatoes, olives, hardboiled egg, and feta.

To taste, season with salt and pepper.

Nutrition:

Calories: 333.7 Cal

Fat: 17 g,

Carbs:3 3.3 g

Protein: 16.3 g

Sugars: 1 g

14. Instant Banana Oatmeal

Preparation Time: 1 Minute

Cooking Time: 2 Minutes

Servings: 1

Ingredients:

1 mashed ripe banana

½ c. water

½ c. quick oats

Directions:

Measure the oats and water into a microwave-safe bowl and stir to combine.

Place bowl in microwave and heat on high for 2 minutes.

Remove bowl from microwave and stir in the mashed banana and enjoy.

Nutrition:

Calories: 243 Cal

Fat: 3 g

Carbs: 50 g

Protein: 6 g

Sugars: 20 g

15. Almond Butter-Banana Smoothie

Preparation Time: 5 Minutes

Cooking Time: 0

Servings: 1

Ingredients:

1 tbsp. almond butter

½ c. ice cubes

½ c. packed spinach

1 peeled and frozen medium banana

1 c. fat-free milk

Directions:

In a powerful blender, blend all ingredients until smooth and creamy.

Serve and enjoy.

Nutrition:

Calories: 293 Cal

Fat:9.8 g

Carbs:42.5 g

Protein:13.5 g

Sugars:12 g

16. Brown Sugar Cinnamon Oatmeal

Preparation Time: 1 Minute

Cooking Time: 3 Minutes

Servings: 4

Ingredients:

½ tsp. ground cinnamon

1 ½ tsps. pure vanilla extract

¼ c. light brown sugar

2 c. low-fat milk

1 1/3 c. quick oats

Directions:

Measure the milk and vanilla into a medium saucepan and bring to a boil over medium-high heat.

Once boiling, reduce heat to medium. Stir in oats, brown sugar, and cinnamon, and cook, stirring, 2–3 minutes.

Serve immediately, sprinkled with additional cinnamon if desired.

Nutrition:

Calories: 208 Cal

Fat:3 g

Carbs:38 g

Protein:8 g

Sugars:15 g

17. Buckwheat Pancakes with Vanilla Almond Milk

Preparation Time: 10 Minutes

Cooking Time: 4 Minutes

Servings: 1

Ingredients:

½ c. unsweetened vanilla almond milk

2-4 packets natural sweetener

1/8 tsp. salt

½ cup buckwheat flour

½ tsp. double-acting baking powder

Directions:

Prepare a nonstick pancake griddle and spray with the cooking spray, place over medium heat.

Whisk together the buckwheat flour, salt, baking powder, and stevia in a small bowl and stir in the almond milk after.

Onto the pan, scoop a large spoonful of batter, cook until bubbles no longer pop on the surface and the entire surface looks dry and (2-4 minutes). Flip and cook for another 2-4 minutes. Repeat with all the remaining batter.

Nutrition:

Calories: 240 Cal Fat:4.5 g

Carbs:2 g Protein:11 g Sugars:17 g

18. Tomato Bruschetta with Basil

Preparation Time: 10 Minutes

Cooking Time: 0

Servings: 8

Ingredients: ½ c. chopped basil

2 minced garlic cloves

1 tbsp. balsamic vinegar 2 tbsps. Olive oil

½ tsp. cracked black pepper

1 sliced whole wheat baguette

8 diced ripe Roma tomatoes

1 tsp. sea salt

Directions:

First, preheat the oven to 375 F.

In a bowl, dice the tomatoes, mix in balsamic vinegar, chopped basil, garlic, salt, pepper, and olive oil, set aside.

Slice the baguette into 16-18 slices and for about 10 minutes, place on a baking pan to bake.

Serve with warm bread slices and enjoy.

For leftovers, store in an airtight container and put in the fridge. Try putting them over grilled chicken, it is amazing!

Nutrition:

Calories: 57 Cal Fat:2.5 g

Carbs:7.9 g Protein:1.4 g Sugars:0.2 g

19. Sweet Corn Muffins

Preparation Time: 5 Minutes

Cooking Time: 15 Minutes

Servings: 1

Ingredients:

1 tbsp. sodium-free baking powder

¾ c. nondairy milk 1 tsp. pure vanilla extract

½ c. sugar 1 c. white whole-wheat flour

1 c. cornmeal   ½ c. canola oil

Directions:

Preheat the oven to 400°F. Line a 12-muffin tin with paper liners and set aside.

Place the cornmeal, flour, sugar, and baking powder into a mixing bowl and whisk well to combine.

Add the nondairy milk, oil, and vanilla and stir just until combined.

Divide the batter evenly between the muffin cups. Place muffin tin on middle rack in oven and bake for 15 minutes.

Remove from oven and place on a wire rack to cool.

Nutrition:

Calories: 203 Cal

Fat:9 g

Carbs:26 g Protein:3 g Sugars:9.5 g

20. Scrambled Eggs with Mushrooms and Spinach

Preparation Time: 5 Minutes

Cooking Time: 10 Minutes

Servings: 1

Ingredients:

2 egg whites

1 slice whole wheat toast

½ c. sliced fresh mushrooms

2 tbsps. Shredded fat free American cheese

Pepper

1 tsp. olive oil

1 c. chopped fresh spinach

1 whole egg

Directions:

On medium high fire, place a nonstick fry pan and add oil. Swirl oil to cover pan and heat for a minute.

Add spinach and mushrooms. Sauté until spinach is wilted, around 2-3 minutes.

Meanwhile, in a bowl whisk well egg, egg whites, and cheese. Season with pepper.

Pour egg mixture into pan and scramble until eggs are cooked through, around 3-4 minutes.

Serve and enjoy with a piece of whole wheat toast.

Nutrition:

Calories: 290.6 Cal

Fat:11.8 g

Carbs:21.8 g

Protein:24.3 g

Sugars:1.4 g

Meat and Poultry Recipes

21. Spicy Habanero and Ground Beef Dinner

Preparation Time: 10 Minutes

Cooking Time: 30 Minutes

Servings: 2

Ingredients: 1/2 teaspoon dried thyme

1/2 teaspoon ground black pepper

1/2 teaspoon dried basil

1 ½ pounds ground chuck

1 teaspoon habanero pepper, minced

1/2 teaspoon ground bay leaf

2 tablespoons tallow, at room temperature

2 ripe Roma tomatoes, crushed

2 shallots, chopped 1 teaspoon fennel seeds

2 garlic cloves, minced

1/4 teaspoon caraway seeds, ground

1/2 cup dry sherry wine

1/2 teaspoon paprika 1/2 teaspoon salt

For Ketogenic Tortillas:

A pinch of table salt 4 egg whites

A pinch of Swerve

1/3 teaspoon baking powder

1/4 cup coconut flour 6 tablespoons water

Directions:

Dissolve the tallow in a wok that is forehead over a normal high heat.

Following the above step, brown the ground chuck for 4 minutes, breaking it with a fork. Include all seasonings along with garlic, shallots, and habanero pepper. After that, keep on cooking for an additional 9 minutes.

Succeeding the above step, stir in the tomatoes and sherry. Then adjust the heat to medium-low, shut the lid, and let it simmer for a longer period of 20 minutes.

In the meantime, prepare the tortillas by mixing the coconut flour, eggs, and baking powder in a container. Add together the salt, water, and Swerve, then mix until everything is well included.

Foreheat a nonstick skillet with a moderate flame. Bake tortillas for a notable time on each side. Again, repeat until there is no more batter. Enjoy ground beef mixture.

Nutrition:

Calories: 361 Cal Protein: 29 g Fat: 21.9 g

Carbs: 6.4 g Sugar: 1.5 g

22. Meatballs with Roasted Peppers and Manchego

Preparation Time: 10 Minutes

Cooking Time 50 Minutes

Servings: 2

Ingredients:

2 leeks, chopped

2 ripe tomatoes, crushed

1 pound ground beef

1 teaspoon lemon thyme

3 garlic cloves

1 egg

3 tablespoons parmesan cheese, grated

1 ½ cups chicken broth

1/2 teaspoon fresh ginger, ground

4 bell peppers, deveined and chopped

2 chipotle peppers, deveined and minced

1/2 cup Manchego cheese, crumbled

Salt and freshly ground black pepper

Directions:

Heat- Broil the peppers for about 20 minutes while turning once or twice). Permit them to stand for about a minimum of 30 minutes to loosen the skin.

Skin the peppers; get rid of stems and seeds; slice chipotle peppers into equal parts and reserve.

In a mixing dish, merge the parmesan, leeks, egg, garlic, salt, pepper, and ground beef. Cook a heavy-bottomed skillet over moderately high heat.

Brown meatballs on all sides for about 10 minutes.

After the above step, make the tomato sauce. Cook the tomatoes, ginger, chicken broth, and lemon thyme in a pan that is preheated over medium-high heat; spice with salt and pepper to taste.

Enable it to boil, reduce the heat to medium. Add meatballs and let them simmer until they are completely cooked, careful stirring.

Serve meatballs with the tomato sauce and roasted peppers. Garnish with crumbled Manchego and serve!

Nutrition:

Calories: 348 Cal

Protein: 42.8 g

Fat: 13.7 g

Carbs: 5.9 g

Sugar: 2.7 g

23. The Best Sloppy Joes Ever

Preparation Time: 10 minutes

Cooking Time: 20 Minutes

Servings: 6

Ingredients: 1 teaspoon deli mustard

Salt and ground pepper, to taste

1 ½ pounds ground chuck

2 teaspoons tallow, room temperature

2 shallots, finely chopped

1 tablespoon coconut vinegar

1 teaspoon chipotle powder

1 teaspoon celery seeds

1/2 cup pureed tomatoes

1 teaspoon garlic, minced

1 teaspoon cayenne pepper

Directions:

Dissolve 1 tablespoon of tallow in a heavy-bottomed skillet using a normal high flame.

After the above, sauté the shallots and garlic till they become tender and aromatic; reserve.

In the same skillet, dissolve another tablespoon of tallow. After that, brown ground chuck, crumbling with a spatula.

Include the vegetables back to the skillet; mix in the remaining ingredients. Set the heat to medium-low; simmer for 20 minutes; stirring every so often.

Enjoy over buns. Bon appétit!

Nutrition:

Calories: 313 Cal

Protein: 26.6 g

Fat: 20.6 g

Carbs: 3.5 g

Sugar: 0.3 g

24. Grilled Rib Eye Steak

Preparation Time: 15 Minutes

Cooking Time: 5 Minutes

Servings: 6

Ingredients:

1 tablespoon Worcestershire sauce

2 tablespoons olive oil

2 tablespoons dry red wine

Celery salt and ground black pepper, to taste

1 tablespoon oyster sauce

2 garlic cloves, smashed

1 thyme sprig, chopped

2 rosemary sprigs, chopped

1 teaspoon dried sage, crushed

1/2 teaspoon chipotle powder

2 pounds rib-eye steaks

Directions:

In a mixing bowl, completely merge oyster sauce and garlic, Worcestershire sauce, thyme, rosemary, salt, sage, chipotle powder, pepper, wine and olive oil.

After that, marinate the rib eye steaks in your refrigerator overnight.

Preheat your grill that is previously lightly greased. Grill rib-eye steaks over direct heat for 4 to 5 minutes on each side for medium-rare. Bon appétit!

Nutrition:

Calories: 314 Cal

Protein: 48.2 g

Fat: 11.4 g

Carbs: 1 g

Sugar: 0.6 g

25. Beef Sausage with Mayo Sauce

Preparation Time: 10 Minutes

Cooking Time: 5 Minutes

Servings: 4

Ingredients:

1 garlic clove, finely minced

2 tablespoons cilantro, minced

1/2 teaspoon dried marjoram

1/2 teaspoon salt

1/3 teaspoon red pepper flakes

1 tablespoon lard, at room temperature

1 red onion, chopped

1 tablespoon tomato puree

1-pound beef sausage, crumbled

For the Sauce:

1 ½ teaspoon mustard

1/4 cup mayonnaise

1 teaspoon cayenne pepper

A pinch of salt

Directions:

Dissolve the lard over medium-high heat. Include the onion and garlic and heat for 2 minutes or till they become tender and fragrant.

Stir in the beef and commence on cooking cook for about 3 minutes longer. Stir in the red pepper, salt, marjoram and cilantro; Heat for 1 additional minute.

After, make the sauce by whisking all the sauce ingredients. Enjoy over low-carb flat bread.

Nutrition:

Calories: 549 Cal Protein: 16.2 g

Fat: 49.3 g Carbs: 4.7 g

Sugar: 2.3 g

26. Slow Cooker Beef Chuck Roast

Preparation Time: 20 Minutes

Cooking Time: 6 Hours

Servings: 8

Ingredients:

1 large-sized white onion, cut into wedges

Salt and pepper to taste

2 rosemary springs 1 thyme sprig

2 tablespoons fresh parsley, chopped

2 tablespoons Worcestershire sauce

3 garlic cloves, minced

2 pounds beef chuck roast

1 cup Provolone, sliced

2 tablespoons olive oil

1/3 cup dry red wine 1/2 cup beef broth

Directions:

Include the beef, garlic, olive oil, onion, rosemary and thyme to your Crock pot.

After the above, include dry red wine, pepper, salt, Worcestershire sauce, beef broth.

Shut the lid and cook on High settings until meat is tender, duration of 6 hours.

Enjoy garnished with fresh parsley and sliced Provolone cheese. Bon appétit!

Nutrition: Calories:519 Cal Protein: 34.4 g

Fat: 39.6 g Carbs: 2.7 gSugar: 1.4 g

27. Finger-Lickin' Good Beef Brisket

Preparation Time: 1 Hour

Cooking Time: 2 Hours and 30 Minutes

Servings: 8

Ingredients: 2 garlic cloves, halved

1 teaspoon shallot powder

1/2 teaspoon freshly ground black pepper

1/4 cup dry red wine 1 teaspoon sea salt

1 tablespoon Dijon mustard

2 pounds beef brisket, trimmed

1 teaspoon dried marjoram

1 teaspoon dried rosemary

Directions:

Begin by preheating an oven to 3750F. Wipe the raw brisket with garlic and Dijon mustard. Now, Peform a dry rub by merging the remaining ingredients. Season the brisket on both sides using the rub. Transfer the wine into the pan. Lay the beef brisket in a baking pan. Roast in the oven for 1 hour. Reduce the temperature of the oven to 3000F; roast for an additional duration of 2 hours 30 minutes.

Now, slice the meat and enjoy with juice from the baking pan. Bon appétit!

Nutrition:

Calories: 219 Cal Protein: 34.6 g Fat: 7.2 g

Carbs: 0.6 g Sugar: 0.1 g

28. Winter Guinness Beef Stew

Preparation Time: 10 Minutes

Cooking Time: 50 Minutes

Servings: 6

Ingredients 1 ½ cups tomato puree

1 cup leeks, chopped

1 bay leaf 1 celery stalk, chopped

3 cups boiling water 1 cup Guinness beer

1/4 cup mint leaves, chopped, to serve

1 tablespoon beef bouillon granules

1 ½ pounds chuck shoulder, cut into bite-size cubes

1 ½ tablespoons avocado oil

1/2 teaspoon caraway seeds

Directions:

Apply heat to the oil in a stockpot over medium-high heat. Now, sauté chuck shoulder cubes till they are browned; reserve. Now, sauté the vegetables in pan drippings for about 8 minutes, stirring every so often. Add the remaining ingredients, leaving out forming leaves, and expose it to a rapid boil. After that, turn the heat to medium-low; allow it simmer for about 50 minutes. Scoop into individual bowls and serve garnished with mint leaves. Bon appétit!

Nutrition: Calories: 444 Cal Protein: 66.3 g Fat: 14.2 g Carbs: 6.1 g Sugar: 2.7 g

29. Greek Prosciutto-Wrapped Meatloaf

Preparation Time: 10 Minutes

Cooking Time:50 Minutes

Servings: 8

Ingredients: 8 slices of prosciutto

2 teaspoons Greek seasoning blend

1/4 cup half-and-half

1/2-pound ground lamb

2 eggs, beaten 1 tablespoon Worcester sauce

3 teaspoons olive oil 2 pounds ground beef

2 shallots, finely chopped

6 ounces feta cheese, crumbled

1 tablespoon brown mustard

1/2 cup chopped Kalamata olives

Directions: Preheat your oven to a 3900F. Heat the oil in a cast-iron skillet that is fore heated using a medium flame. Sauté the shallot until it gets soft and lightly browned. In a large mixing container, completely merge the remaining ingredients, leaving out prosciutto. Add sautéed onion and stir well. Shape the merge substance into a meatloaf. Wrap the meatloaf in the slices of prosciutto and move it to a baking pan. Close it with a piece of aluminum foil. Bake for 40 minutes. Dispose of the foil and bake for an extra 10 to 13 minutes. Bon appétit!

Nutrition: Calories: 442 Cal Protein: 56.3 g Fat: 20.6 g Carbs: 4.9 g Sugar: 1 g

30. Greek-Style Cold Beef Salad

Preparation Time: 15 Minutes

Cooking Time: 3 Minutes

Servings: 6

Ingredients:

1 orange bell pepper, thinly sliced

1 green bell pepper, thinly sliced

1 tablespoon fresh lemon juice

Salt and ground black pepper, to your liking

1 cup grape tomatoes, halved

1 tablespoon soy sauce

1 ½ pounds beef rump steak

1/2 teaspoon dried oregano

1 head of butter lettuce, leaves separated

1 red onion, peeled and thinly sliced

2 cucumbers, thinly sliced

1/4 cup extra-virgin olive oil

Directions:

In a salad container, toss the onions, cucumbers, tomato, bell pepper, and butter lettuce leaves.

Fore heat a barbecue grill; heat the steak for 3 minutes per side. After that, thinly slice steak across the grain.

Include the slices of meat to the salad.

Prepare the dressing by whisking the oregano, salt, pepper, lemon juice, olive oil and soy sauce.

Dress the salad and enjoy well-chilled.

Nutrition:

Calories: 315 Protein: 37.5g

Fat: 13.8g Carbs: 6.4g Sugar: 2.4g

31. Slow Cooked Chicken Curry

Preparation Time: 10 Minutes

Cooking Time: 5 Hours

Servings: 4

Ingredients: 2 sweet potatoes, cubed

3 chicken breasts, boneless, skinless and chopped

1 red bell pepper, chopped

1 small yellow onion, chopped

2 cups coconut milk   2 cups chicken stock

1 teaspoon ground cumin

3 tablespoons curry powder

2 tablespoons chopped cilantro

Salt and cayenne pepper to the taste

Directions:

In your slow cooker, mix the chicken the sweet potatoes, bell pepper, onion, stock, milk, cumin, curry powder, salt and cayenne.

Cover and cook on Low for 5 hours then divide into bowls, sprinkle the cilantro on top and serve.

Enjoy!

Nutrition:

Calories: 280 Cal Fat: 13 g

Fiber: 7 g Carbs: 8 g Protein: 15 g

32. Cumin Chicken Mix

Preparation Time: 2 Hours

Cooking Time: 25 Minutes

Servings: 4

Ingredients:

4 garlic cloves, minced

2 pounds chicken thighs, skinless and boneless

4 tablespoons extra-virgin olive oil

4 tablespoons chopped cilantro

2 tablespoons lime juice

A pinch of salt and black pepper

2 tablespoons olive oil

1 teaspoon cumin, ground

1 teaspoon red chili flakes

Lime wedges for serving

Directions:

In a bowl, whisk the olive oil with salt, pepper, cilantro, garlic, lime juice, cumin and chili flakes. Add the chicken, toss, cover and leave aside for 2 hours. Heat up a pan with the oil over medium-high heat, add chicken, cook for 3 minutes on each side and transfer to a baking dish. Cook in the oven at 375 degrees F for 20 minutes then divide between plates and serve with lime wedges on the side.

Enjoy!

Nutrition:

Calories: 200 Cal

Fat: 10 g Fiber: 1 g

Carbs: 12 g Protein: 24 g

33. Rosemary Chicken Thighs

Preparation Time: 10 Minutes

Cooking Time: 40 Minutes

Servings: 2

Ingredients:

14 ounces chicken thighs, bone-in

1 tablespoon lemon juice

1 teaspoon chili powder

A pinch of salt and black pepper

1 tablespoon fresh minced ginger

1 tablespoon olive oil

4 onions, chopped

2 rosemary springs, chopped

Directions:

In a bowl, mix chili powder with lemon juice and ginger. Add the chicken, rub it with this mix and then let sit for 10 minutes. Heat up a pan with the oil over medium-high heat, add the marinated chicken pieces and cook for 3 minutes on each side. Add rosemary, onions, salt and pepper. Reduce heat to medium, cover pan, cook for 25 minutes. Divide between plates and serve.

Enjoy!

Nutrition:

Calories 210 g

Fat 8 g

Fiber 9 g

Carbs 12 g

Protein 17 g

34. Turkey Stew

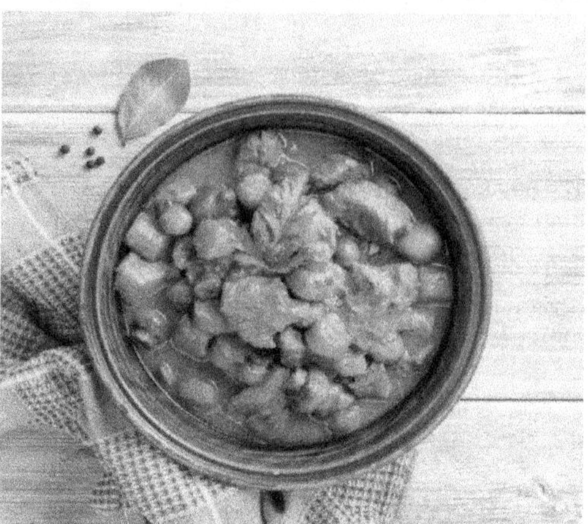

Preparation Time: 10 Minutes

Cooking Time: 1 Hour And 20 Minutes

Servings: 6

Ingredients:

3 teaspoons olive oil

1 green bell pepper, chopped

1 pound ground turkey meat

1 tablespoons garlic, minced

1 yellow onion, chopped

1 teaspoon ground ancho chilies

1 tablespoon chili powder

2 teaspoons ground cumin

8 ounces canned green chilies and juice, chopped

8 ounces tomato paste

15 ounces canned tomatoes, chopped

2 cups veggie stock

A pinch of salt and black pepper

Directions:

Heat up a pan with 2 teaspoons oil over medium heat, add turkey, stir, brown well on all sides and transfer to a pot. Heat up the pan with the rest of the oil over medium heat and add onion and green bell pepper. Stir and cook for 3 minutes. Add garlic, chili powder, ancho chili powder, salt, pepper and cumin, stir and cook for 2 more minutes. Transfer this to the pot with the turkey meat, add chilies and juice, tomato sauce, chopped tomatoes, stock, salt and pepper. Stir, bring to a boil, cover the pot and cook for 1 hour. Divide into bowls and serve.

Enjoy!

Nutrition:

Calories: 327

Fat: 8

Fiber: 13

Carbs: 24

Protein: 27

35. Chicken and Mushroom Salad

Preparation Time: 10 Minutes

Cooking Time: 0 Minutes

Servings: 4

Ingredients:

1 yellow onion, chopped

12 ounces canned mushrooms, drained and chopped

2 garlic cloves, minced

2 teaspoons chopped rosemary

3 cups chicken, already cooked and shredded

2 cups baby spinach

Salt and black pepper to the tastes

A splash of balsamic vinegar

A drizzle of olive oil

Directions:

In a bowl, mix the mushrooms with the chicken, onion, garlic, rosemary, spinach, salt, pepper, vinegar and oil, toss and serve.

Enjoy!

Nutrition:

Calories: 210 Cal Fat: 5 g

Fiber: 8 g Carbs: 15 g

Protein:11 g

36. Chicken Roast

Preparation Time: 10 Minutes

Cooking Time: 1 Hour And 10 Minutes

Servings: 4

Ingredients:

1 whole chicken

A pinch of salt and black pepper

2 tablespoons olive oil

2 green onions, chopped

1 cup chicken stock

2 teaspoons lemon juice

2 teaspoons chopped rosemary

Directions:

Place chicken in a roasting pan, add salt, pepper, oil, green onions, stock, lemon juice and rosemary. Toss the ingredients together, place in the oven and bake at 450 degrees F for 1 hour. Slice the meat, divide it between plates and serve with cooking juices drizzled on top.

Enjoy!

Nutrition:

Calories: 495 Cal Fat: 8 g

Fiber: 4 g Carbs: 10 g

Protein: 27 g

37. Ginger Chicken Thighs

Preparation Time: 12 Hours

Cooking Time: 1 Hour

Servings: 4

Ingredients:

8 chicken thighs, bone in and skin on

A pinch of sea salt and black pepper

1 tablespoon apple cider vinegar

3 tablespoons chopped onion

1 tablespoon fresh grated ginger

½ teaspoon dried thyme

¾ cup apple juice

½ cup maple syrup

Directions:

In a bowl, combine chicken thighs with salt, pepper, vinegar, onion, ginger, thyme, apple juice and maple syrup. Cover and keep in the fridge for 12 hours to marinate. Transfer this whole mix to a baking dish, cover dish, bake in the oven at 400 degrees F for 1 hour. Divide the meat and sauce between plates and serve.

Enjoy!

Nutrition: Calories 274

Fat 6 Fiber 8

Carbs 14 Protein 12

38. Thai Chicken Thighs

Preparation Time: 10 Minutes

Cooking Time: 6 Hours And 10 Minutes

Servings: 6

Ingredients:

4 pounds chicken thighs, skin-on and bone-in

1 bunch green onions, chopped

½ cup Thai sweet chili sauce

Directions:

Heat up a pan over medium-high heat, add chicken thighs and brown them for 5 minutes on each side. Transfer the chicken to your slow cooker, add green onions and chili sauce, cover and cook on Low for 6 hours. Divide between plates and serve.

Enjoy!

Nutrition:

Calories: 260 Cal

Fat: 4 g

Fiber: 2 g

Carbs: 12 g

Protein: 14 g

39. Chicken with Parsley Sauce

Preparation Time: 30 Minutes

Cooking Time: 40 Minutes

Servings: 6

Ingredients:

1 cup chopped parsley

1 teaspoon dried oregano

½ cup olive oil

¼ cup vegetable stock

4 garlic cloves

A pinch of salt and black pepper

12 chicken thighs

Directions:

In your food processor, mix parsley with oregano, garlic, salt, oil and the stock. Pulse well until smooth. In a bowl, mix the chicken with the parsley sauce and toss, cover and keep in the fridge for 30 minutes. Heat up your kitchen grill over medium heat and place the chicken pieces on the grill. Close the lid and cook for 20 minutes. Flip the chicken and cook for 20 minutes more. Divide between plates and serve with the parsley sauce on top.

Enjoy!

Nutrition:

Calories: 254 Cal Fat: 3 g Fiber: 3 g

Carbs: 7 g Protein: 12 g

40. Chicken and Lentil Casserole

Preparation Time: 10 Minutes

Cooking Time: 1 Hour And 40 Minutes

Servings: 8

Ingredients:

1½ cups green lentils

3 cups clean chicken stock

2-pound chicken breasts, skinless, boneless and cubed

A pinch of sea salt and cayenne pepper

3 teaspoons ground cumin

Cooking spray

5 garlic cloves, minced

1 yellow onion, chopped

2 red bell peppers, chopped

14 ounces canned tomatoes, chopped

2 cups corn

2 tablespoons chopped jalapeno pepper

1 tablespoon garlic powder

1 cup chopped parsley

Directions:

Put the stock in a pot, add a pinch of salt and the lentils. Stir, bring to a boil over medium heat, cover and simmer for 35 minutes. Heat up a pan with some cooking spray over medium-high heat and add the chicken, season with salt, cayenne pepper and 1 teaspoon cumin. Cook for 5 minutes on each side then transfer to a bowl. Heat up the pan again over medium heat, add bell peppers, garlic, onion, tomatoes, salt, cayenne and 1 teaspoon cumin. Stir, cook for 7 minutes and transfer to the bowl with the chicken. Drain the lentils, add them to the bowl with the meat and then add jalapeno pepper, garlic powder, the rest of the cumin, corn and parsley. Toss, transfer the whole mix to a baking dish and place in the oven at 350 degrees F and bake for 50 minutes. Divide between plates and serve.

Enjoy!

Nutrition:

Calories: 244

Fat: 11

Fiber: 4

Carbs: 10

Protein: 13

Seafood Recipes

41. Poached Halibut and Mushrooms

Preparation Time: 5 Minutes

Cooking Time: 30 Minutes

Servings: 8

Ingredients: 1/8 teaspoon sesame oil

2 pounds halibut, cut into bite-sized pieces

1 teaspoon fresh lemon juice

½ teaspoon soy sauce

4 cups mushrooms, sliced   ¼ cup water

Salt and pepper to taste   ¾ cup green onions

Directions:

Place a heavy bottomed pot on medium high fire.

Add all ingredients and mix well.

Cover and bring to a boil. Once boiling, lower fire to a simmer. Cook for 25 minutes.

Adjust seasoning to taste.

Serve and enjoy.

Nutrition:

Calories: 217 Cal Fat 15.8 g Carbs: 1.1 g

Protein: 16.5 g Fiber: 0.4 g

42. Halibut Stir Fry

Preparation Time: 5 Minutes

Cooking Time: 20 Minutes

Servings: 6

Ingredients: 2 pounds halibut fillets

2 tbsp olive oil   ½ cup fresh parsley

1 onion, sliced   2 stalks celery, chopped

2 tablespoons capers

4 cloves of garlic minced

Salt and pepper to taste

Directions:

Place a heavy bottomed pot on high fire and heat for 2 minutes. Add oil and heat for 2 more minutes.

Stir in garlic and onions. Sauté for 5 minutes. Add remaining ingredients, except for parsley and stir fry for 10 minutes or until fish is cooked.

Adjust seasoning to taste and serve with a sprinkle of parsley.

Nutrition:

Calories 331 Cal Fat 26 g Carbs 2 g

Protein 22 g Fiber 0.5 g

43. Steamed Garlic-Dill Halibut

Preparation Time: 5 Minutes

Cooking Time: 25 Minutes

Servings: 4

Ingredients:

1-pound halibut fillet

1 lemon, freshly squeezed

Salt and pepper to taste

1 teaspoon garlic powder

1 tablespoon dill weed, chopped

Directions:

Place a large pot on medium fire and fill up to 1.5-inches of water. Place a trivet inside pot.

In a baking dish that fits inside your large pot, add all ingredients and mix well. Cover dish with foil. Place the dish on top of the trivet inside the pot.

Cover pot and steam fish for 15 minutes.

Let fish rest for at least 10 minutes before removing from pot.

Serve and enjoy.

Nutrition:

Calories: 270 Cal

Fat: 6.5 g

Carbs: 3.9 g

Protein: 47.8 g Fiber: 2.1 g

44. Italian Halibut Chowder

Preparation Time: 5 Minutes

Cooking Time: 20 Minutes

Servings: 8

Ingredients:

2 tablespoons olive oil

1 onion, chopped

3 stalks of celery, chopped

3 cloves of garlic, minced

2 ½ pounds halibut steaks, cubed

1 red bell pepper, seeded and chopped

1 cup tomato juice

½ cup apple juice, organic and unsweetened

½ teaspoon dried basil

1/8 teaspoon dried thyme

Salt and pepper to taste

Directions:

Place a heavy bottomed pot on medium high fire and heat pot for 2 minutes. Add oil and heat for a minute.

Sauté the onion, celery and garlic until fragrant.

Stir in the halibut steaks and bell pepper. Sauté for 3 minutes.

Pour in the rest of the ingredients and mix well.

Cover and bring to a boil. Once boiling, lower fire to a simmer and simmer for 10 minutes.

Adjust seasoning to taste.

Serve and enjoy.

Nutrition:

Calories: 318 Cal Fat: 23g Carbs: 6g

Protein: 21g Fiber: 1g

45. Stuffed Salmon

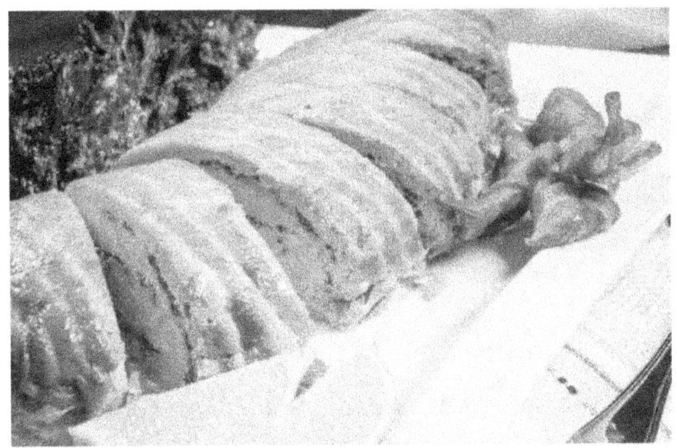

Preparation Time: 10 Minutes

Cooking Time: 20 Minutes

Servings: 2

Ingredients:

2 salmon fillets

4 teaspoons olive oil

5 ounces shrimp, peeled, deveined and chopped

6 mushrooms, chopped

3 green onions, chopped

2 cups baby spinach

¼ cup avocado mayonnaise

¼ teaspoon ground nutmeg

¼ cup chopped walnuts, toasted

A pinch of salt and black pepper

Directions:

Heat up a pan with half of the oil over medium-high heat, add mushrooms, onions, salt and pepper, stir and cook for 4 minutes. Add walnuts, spinach and shrimp then stir and cook for 4 minutes. Remove from the heat and mix with the nutmeg and mayo. Make an incision lengthwise in each salmon fillet then season with salt and pepper and stuff the salmon with the shrimp mix. Heat up a pan with the rest of the oil over medium-high heat, add stuffed salmon, skin side down and cook for 2 minutes. Reduce the heat, cover, cook the fish for 10 minutes. Divide between plates and serve.

Enjoy!

Nutrition:

Calories: 250 Cal

Fat: 10 g

Fiber: 3 g

Carbs: 7 g

Protein: 20 g

46. Mustard Crusted Salmon

Preparation Time: 10 Minutes

Cooking Time: 22 Minutes

Servings: 2

Ingredients:

2 salmon fillets, boneless

A pinch of salt and black pepper

4 tablespoons mustard

2 tablespoons coconut oil

Directions:

Season salmon with salt and pepper and brush it with the mustard on both sides. Heat up a pan with the oil over medium-high heat, place salmon flesh side down and cook for 3 minutes on each side. Transfer to a baking dish and place in the oven at 425 degrees F to bake for 15 minutes then serve with a side salad.

Enjoy!

Nutrition:

Calories 240 Cal

Fat 7 g

Fiber 6 g

Carbs 8 g

Protein 14 g

47. Dill Haddock

Preparation Time: 10 minutes

Cooking Time: 30 minutes

Servings: 4

Ingredients:

1-pound haddock fillets

3 teaspoons veggie stock

2 tablespoons lemon juice

Salt and black pepper to the taste

2 tablespoons mayonnaise

2 teaspoons chopped dill

A drizzle of olive oil

Directions:

Grease a baking dish with the oil, add the fish, also add stock mixed with lemon juice, salt, pepper, mayo and dill. Toss a bit and place in the oven at 350 degrees F to bake for 30 minutes. Divide between plates and serve.

Enjoy!

Nutrition:

Calories: 214

Fat: 12 Cal

Fiber: 4 g

Carbs: 7 g

Protein: 17 g

48. Trout and Salsa

Preparation Time: 10 Minutes

Cooking Time: 16 Minutes

Servings: 2

Ingredients: 2 trout fillets, boneless

½ cup chopped yellow onion

4 teaspoons olive oil

1 teaspoon minced garlic

1 green bell pepper, chopped

½ cup canned tomato salsa

2 tablespoons kalamata olives, pitted and chopped

¼ cup chicken stock

A pinch of salt and black pepper

Directions:

Heat up a pan with 2 teaspoons oil over medium heat, add bell pepper and onion then stir and cook for 3 minutes. Add garlic, stock, olives and salsa, stir, cook for 5 minutes and transfer to a bowl. Heat up the pan again with the rest of the oil over medium heat, add fish, season with salt and pepper and cook for 2 minutes on each side. Transfer to a baking dish, pour the salsa over the fish and place in the oven to bake at 425 degrees F for 6 minutes. Divide between plates and serve.

Enjoy!

Nutrition: Calories: 200 Cal

Fat: 5 g Fiber: 6 g Carbs: 12 g Protein: 12 g

49. Salmon Soup

Preparation Time: 10 Minutes

Cooking Time: 30 Minutes

Servings: 4

Ingredients:

1 red sweet bell pepper, chopped

2 green bell peppers, chopped

3 cups chicken stock

1 tablespoon olive oil

4 celery stick, chopped

1 brown onion, chopped

4 wild salmon fillets, skinless, boneless and cubed

A pinch of sea salt and black pepper

Directions:

Heat up a pot with the oil over medium-high heat, add the onion, stir and cook for 3 minutes. Add the red and green bell pepper, stir and cook for 3 minutes more. Add the celery, salmon, salt, pepper and the stock. Toss a bit then bring to a simmer, reduce heat to medium and cook for 20 minutes. Divide into bowls and serve.

Enjoy!

Nutrition:

Calories: 265 Cal Fat: 7 g

Fiber: 5 g Carbs: 15 g Protein: 16 g

50. Shrimp Cakes

Preparation Time: 10 Minutes

Cooking Time: 10 Minutes

Servings: 24

Ingredients:

½ pound tiger shrimp, peeled, deveined and chopped

A pinch of sea salt and black pepper

2 tablespoons olive oil

½ pound ground pork

1 egg, whisked

2 tablespoons coconut flour

2 tablespoons chicken stock

1 teaspoon coconut aminos

1 green onion stalk, chopped

1 teaspoon fresh grated ginger

Directions:

In a bowl, mix the shrimp with the pork, salt, pepper, egg, stock, aminos, onion, ginger and flour. Stir well and shape medium cakes out of this mix. Heat up a pan with the oil over medium-high heat, add the cakes and cook for 5 minutes on each side. Divide between plates and serve with a side salad.

Enjoy!

Nutrition: Calories 281 Cal

Fat 8 g Fiber 7 g Carbs 19 g Protein 8 g

51. Italian Calamari

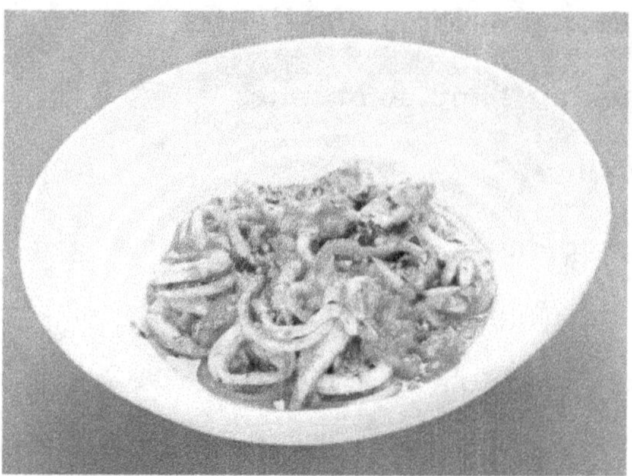

Preparation Time: 10 Minutes

Cooking Time: 30 Minutes

Servings: 6

Ingredients:

15 ounces canned tomatoes, chopped

1 ½ pounds calamari, cleaned, tentacles separated and cut into thin strips

1 garlic clove, minced

½ cup veggie stock

1 bunch chopped parsley

A pinch red pepper flakes

Juice of lemon

A drizzle of olive oil

A pinch of sea salt and black pepper

Directions:

Heat up a pan with the oil over medium-high heat, add the garlic and pepper flakes, stir and cook for 2-3 minutes. Add calamari, stir and cook for 3 minutes more. Add tomatoes, stock, lemon juice, salt and pepper, bring to a simmer then reduce heat to medium and cook for 25 minutes. Add the parsley, stir, divide into bowls and serve.

Enjoy!

Nutrition: Calories 228 Cal

Fat 2 g Fiber 4 g

Carbs 11 g Protein 39 g

52. Chili Snapper

Preparation Time: 10 Minutes

Cooking Time: 20 Minutes

Servings: 2

Ingredients:

2 red snapper fillets, boneless and skinless

3 tablespoons chili paste

A pinch of sea salt and black pepper

1 tablespoon coconut aminos

1 garlic clove, minced

½ teaspoon fresh grated ginger

2 teaspoons sesame seeds, toasted

2 tablespoons olive oil

1 green onion, chopped

2 tablespoons chicken stock

Directions:

Heat up a pan with the oil over medium-high heat, add the ginger, onion and the garlic, stir and cook for 2 minutes. Add chili paste, aminos, salt, pepper and the stock, stir and cook for 3 minutes more. Add the fish fillets, toss gently and cook for 5-6 minutes on each side. Divide between plates, sprinkle sesame seeds on top and serve.

Enjoy!

Nutrition: Calories 261

Fat: 10 g Fiber: 7 g

Carbs: 15 g Protein:16 g

53. Thai Cod

Preparation Time: 10 Minutes

Cooking Time: 10 Minutes

Servings: 2

Ingredients:

1 tablespoon coconut aminos

1 cup coconut milk

1 tablespoon Thai curry paste

A drizzle of olive oil

Zest of 1 lime

Juice of ½ lime

1 tablespoon fresh grated ginger

1 teaspoon garlic, minced

2 cod fillets, boneless

1 tablespoon chopped cilantro

Directions:

In a bowl, whisk the aminos with coconut cream, curry paste, lime zest and juice, ginger and garlic. Add the cod, toss to cover and set aside for 10 minutes to marinate. Heat up a pan with a drizzle of oil over medium heat, add the cod, cook for 5 minutes on each side, divide between plates and sprinkle cilantro on top then serve.

Enjoy!

Nutrition:

Calories: 271 Cal Fat 4 g

Fiber 6 g Carbs 14 g Protein 7 g

54. Cod and Peas

Preparation Time: 10 Minutes

Cooking Time: 15 Minutes

Servings: 4

Ingredients:

10 ounces peas, blanched

1 tablespoon chopped parsley

A drizzle of olive oil

4 cod fillets, boneless

1 teaspoon dried oregano

2 ounces veggie stock

2 garlic cloves, minced

1 teaspoon smoked paprika

A pinch of sea salt and black pepper

Directions:

Put parsley, paprika, oregano, stock and garlic in your food processor and blend really well. Heat up a pan with the oil over medium-high heat, add the cod, season with salt and pepper and cook for 4 minutes on each side. Add the peas and the parsley, mix and cook for 5 minutes more. Divide everything between plates and serve.

Enjoy!

Nutrition:

Calories: 271 Cal Fat: 4 g

Fiber: 6 g Carbs: 14 g Protein: 15 g

55. Salmon and Scallions

Preparation Time: 10 Minutes

Cooking Time: 20 Minutes

Servings: 4

Ingredients:

4 medium salmon fillets, boneless

4 scallions, chopped

2 tablespoons olive oil

Zest of 1 lemon

1 teaspoon white vinegar

¼ cup chopped dill

¼ cup chicken stock

A pinch of sea salt and black pepper

Directions:

Heat up a pan with half of the oil over medium-high heat, add the salmon, season with salt and pepper then cook for 6 minutes on each side and divide between plates. Heat up another pan with the rest of the oil over medium-high heat. Add scallions, stir and cook for 2 minutes. Add lemon zest, vinegar, dill, stock, salt and pepper. Stir and cook for 5 minutes more, pour over the salmon and serve.

Enjoy!

Nutrition:

Calories 300 Cal Fat: 4 g

Fiber: 8 g Carbs: 14 g Protein: 17 g

2 cups baby carrots

1 tablespoon lime juice

A pinch of sea salt and black pepper

Directions:

In a bowl, mix the cinnamon with half of the oil, salt and pepper then rub the salmon with this mix. Place the salmon on the preheated grill over medium-high heat, cook for 5 minutes on each side and divide between plates. Heat up a pan with the rest of the oil over medium-high heat and add the carrots, lime juice, salt and pepper. Toss and cook for 5-6 minutes then divide next to the salmon and serve.

Enjoy!

Nutrition:

Calories: 371

Fat: 26 Fiber: 2

Carbs: 6 Protein: 22

56. Salmon and Carrots

Preparation Time: 10 Minutes

Cooking Time: 15 Minutes

Servings: 2

Ingredients:

1 tablespoon ground cinnamon

2 tablespoon olive oil

2 salmon fillets, bone-in

57. Chinese Mackerel

Preparation Time: 10 Minutes

Cooking Time: 30 Minutes

Servings: 4

Ingredients: 1 garlic clove, minced

1 shallot, chopped   1 cup chicken stock

2 pounds mackerel, skinless, boneless and cubed

1 small ginger piece, chopped

1 yellow onion, chopped

2 celery stalks, chopped

1 teaspoon hot mustard

1 tablespoon rice vinegar

A pinch of black pepper

A drizzle of olive oil

Directions:

Heat up a pan with the oil over medium-high heat, add the mackerel, season with black pepper and cook for 4 minutes. Add the garlic, shallot, onion, ginger and celery, toss and cook for 4 minutes more, flipping the fish as well. Add stock, mustard and vinegar, toss gently and cook for 20 minutes over medium heat. Divide into bowls and serve.

Enjoy!

Nutrition: Calories: 261 Cal Fat: 4 g

Fiber: 8 g Carbs: 14 g Protein: 7 g

58. Lemony Mackerel

Preparation Time: 10 Minutes

Cooking Time: 15 Minutes

Servings: 4

Ingredients:

Juice of 1 lemon

Zest of 1 lemon

4 mackerels

1 tablespoon minced chives

A pinch of sea salt and black pepper

2 tablespoons olive oil

Directions:

Heat up a pan with the oil over medium-high heat, add the mackerel and cook for 6 minutes on each side. Add the lemon zest, lemon juice, chives, salt and pepper then cook for 2 more minutes on each side. Divide everything between plates and serve.

Enjoy!

Nutrition:

Calories: 289 Cal

Fat :20 g

Fiber: 0 g

Carbs: 1 g

Protein: 21 g

59. French Seafood Stew

Preparation Time: 10 Minutes

Cooking Time: 55 Minutes

Servings: 6

Ingredients: 1 fennel bulb, sliced

2 thyme springs, chopped

1 bay leaf

¾ cup olive oil

2 shallots, chopped

2 yellow onions, sliced

3 garlic cloves, minced

2 tomatoes, chopped

1-pound sea bass, skinless, boneless and cubed

1-pound snapper fillets, skinless, boneless and cubed

1-pound shrimp, peeled and deveined

A pinch of salt and black pepper

Directions:

Heat up a pot with the oil over medium-high heat, add shallot, onions and garlic and stir then cook for 4 minutes. Add fennel, thyme, tomatoes, bay leaf, salt and pepper, stir and cook for 5 minutes more. Add the fish and the shrimp, toss and cook for 5 minutes. Add water to cover everything and a little more salt and pepper then bring to a boil over medium heat, cover the pot and cook for 40 minutes stirring often. Remove the bay leaf then divide into bowls and serve.

Enjoy!

Nutrition:

Calories: 251 Cal

Fat: 4 g Fiber: 6 g

Carbs: 14 g Protein: 7 g

60. Scallops Stew

Preparation Time: 10 Minutes

Cooking Time: 20 Minutes

Servings: 4

Ingredients:

2 leeks, chopped

2 tablespoons olive oil

1 teaspoon chopped jalapeno

2 teaspoons chopped garlic

A pinch of salt and black pepper

¼ teaspoon ground cinnamon

1 carrot, chopped

1 teaspoon ground cumin

1½ cups chopped tomatoes

1 cup veggie stock

1-pound shrimp, peeled and deveined

1-pound sea scallops

2 tablespoons chopped cilantro

Directions:

Heat up a pot with the oil over medium heat, add garlic and leeks, stir and cook for 7 minutes. Add jalapeno, salt, pepper, cayenne, carrots, cinnamon and cumin, stir and cook for 5 more minutes. Add tomatoes, stock, shrimp and scallops, stir, cook for 6 more minutes then divide into bowls, sprinkle cilantro on top and serve.

Enjoy!

Nutrition:

Calories: 251 Cal

Fat :4 g

Fiber: 4 g

Carbs: 11 g

Protein: 17 g

Beans and Grains Recipes

61. Baked Beans and Rice

Preparation Time: 10 minutes

Cooking Time: 45 minutes

Servings 6

Ingredients:

1 ½ cups cooked brown rice

1 15-oz can no-salt added black beans, drained and rinsed

1 cup chopped poblano pepper

1 cup chopped red bell pepper

1 cup frozen yellow corn

1 cup shredded reduced fat Monterey Jack cheese

1 lb. skinless, boneless chicken breast cut into bite sized pieces

1 tbsp chili powder

1 tbsp cumin

2 14.5-oz cans no salt added tomatoes, diced or crushed

4 garlic cloves, crushed

Directions:

With cooking spray, grease a 3-quart shallow casserole and preheat oven to 400oF.

Spread cooked brown rice in bottom of casserole.

Layer chicken on top of brown rice.

Mix well garlic, seasonings, peppers, corn, beans and tomatoes in a medium bowl.

Evenly spread bean mixture on top of chicken.

Sprinkle cheese on top of beans and pop into the oven.

Bake for 45 minutes, remove from oven and serve.

Nutrition:

Calories 291

Fat 8g

Carbs 27g

Protein 27g

Fiber 5g

62. Roasted Grain-Veggie Salad

Preparation Time: 15 minutes

Cooking Time: 45 minutes

Servings 6

Ingredients:

1 cup millet

1 cup quinoa

1/8 teaspoon curry powder (optional)

4 cups chicken stock or vegetable stock (more, as needed)

1/4 cup sun-dried tomatoes (dried in a package, not in oil)

1/2 cup boiling purified water

1/2 cup shredded zucchini

1/2 cup shredded yellow summer squash

1/4 cup minced red bell pepper

1/4 cup chopped scallions or green onions

Salt to taste

Directions:

Toast the millet and quinoa in a large saucepan set over low heat, stirring it constantly until it turns a light brown color, less than 1 minute.

Stir in the curry powder until it is blended in. Remove from heat and let cool for 5 minutes.

Add the chicken or vegetable stock and bring to a boil.

Reduce heat, cover, and simmer. Check after 20 minutes.

If the stock has boiled away, add a little more. Cook until the grains have absorbed all the liquid, about 25 minutes in all.

Meanwhile, soak the dried tomatoes in the boiling water for 15 minutes.

Drain them in a colander set over a bowl to reserve the liquid, then chop them.

Mix the tomatoes, reserved liquid, zucchini, yellow squash, red pepper, and scallions or green onions together in a small skillet set over low heat and cook until most of the liquid is absorbed.

Pour into the cooked grain and toss until everything is completely mixed together. Taste and add salt if you think it is needed.

Fluff with a fork and serve.

Nutrition:

Calories 153.9

Fat 6.2g

Carbs 22.7g

Protein 4.2g

Fiber 3.0g

63. Tandoori Cauliflower-Rice Bowl

Preparation Time: 10 minutes

Cooking Time: 50 minutes

Servings 4

Ingredients:

2 tablespoons chopped fresh cilantro

1 English cucumber, seeded and diced

Lemon wedges, for serving

2 boneless, skinless chicken breasts (about 12 ounces total)

2 cups plain whole-fat yogurt

2 tablespoons lemon juice

3 teaspoons curry powder

2 teaspoons finely grated ginger

1 1/2 teaspoons finely grated garlic

Kosher salt

4 cups bite-size cauliflower florets (about 8 ounces)

1 tablespoon olive oil 2 ¾ cups water

2 cups basmati or other long-grain rice

1/4 cup tomato paste 4 wide strips lemon zest

Directions:

Slice chicken breasts into two thin slices.

In a bowl whisk well 2 tsp salt, ½ tsp grated garlic, 1 tsp grated ginger, 2 tsp curry powder, 1 tbsp lemon juice, and 1 cup yogurt. Divide yogurt mixture into two bowls. In one bowl, marinate chicken breast. In the other bowl, marinate cauliflower. Set aside for 15 minutes.

In large saucepan on medium high fire heat oil for 3 minutes.

Stir in rice and remaining garlic and ginger. Cook for a minute.

Stir in tomato paste and mix well. Add water, 1 tbsp salt, and lemon zest.

Bring to a boil. Once boiling, lower fire to a simmer, cover pan, and cook for 20 minutes.

Turn off fire, fluff rice, cover and let it rest for 5 minutes. Discard lemon zest.

In a medium bowl, mix well 1 tsp salt, 1 tbsp lemon juice, 1 cup yogurt, cucumber, 1 tbsp cilantro.

Preheat broiler and place rack on the topmost part of oven. Lightly grease baking sheets with cooking spray and lay marinated chicken on one sheet and on the other sheet evenly spread cauliflower.

Broil for 12 minutes.

Divide rice into four bowls. Top with ¼ of each of the cucumber sauce, cauliflower, and chicken. Garnish with remaining cilantro and lemon wedges.

Nutrition:

Calories 383 Fat 11g Carbs 44g

Protein 29g Fiber 6g,

64. Roasted Vegetables with Polenta

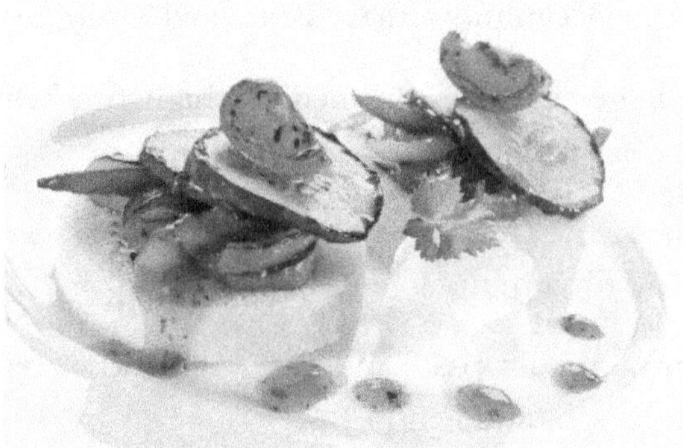

Preparation Time: 10 minutes

Cooking Time: 35 minutes

Servings 6

Ingredients:

2 tsp oregano

10 ripe olives, chopped

6 dry-packed sun-dried tomatoes, soaked in water to rehydrate, drained and chopped

2 plum or Roma tomatoes, sliced

10-oz frozen spinach, thawed

¼ tsp cracked black pepper

2 tsp trans-free margarine

1 ½ cups coarse polenta

6 cups water

2 tbsp + 1 tsp extra virgin olive oil

1 sweet red pepper, seeded, cored and cut into chunks

6 medium mushrooms, sliced

1 small green zucchini, cut into ¼-inch slices

1 small yellow zucchini, cut into ¼-inch slices

1 small eggplant, peeled and cut into ¼-inch slices

Directions:

Grease a baking sheet and a 12-inch circle baking dish, position oven rack 4-inches away from heat source and preheat broiler.

With 1 tbsp olive oil, brush red pepper, mushrooms, zucchini and eggplant. Place in prepared baking sheet in a single layer. Pop in the broiler and broil under low setting.

Turn and brush again with oil the veggies after 5 minutes. Continue broiling until veggies are slightly browned and tender.

Wash and drain spinach. Set aside.

Preheat oven to 350oF.

Bring water to a boil in a medium saucepan.

Whisk in polenta and lower fire to a simmer. For 5 minutes, cook and stir.

Once polenta no longer sticks to pan, add 1/8 tsp pepper and margarine. Mix well and turn off fire.

Evenly spread polenta on base of prepped baking dish. Brush tops with olive oil and for ten minutes bake in the oven.

When done, remove polenta from oven and keep warm.

With paper towels remove excess water from spinach. Layer spinach on top of polenta followed by sliced tomatoes, olives, sun-dried tomatoes, and roasted veggies. Season with remaining pepper and bake for another 10 minutes.

Remove from oven, cut into equal servings and enjoy.

Nutrition:

Calories 135

Fat 2g

Carbs 27g

Protein 5g

Fiber: 6g

65. Cherries and Quinoa

Preparation Time: 5 Minutes

Cooking Time: 10 Minutes

Servings 1

Ingredients:

1 tsp honey – optional

¼ tsp ground cinnamon

½ tsp vanilla extract

½ cup dried unsweetened cherries

½ cup dry quinoa

1 cup water

Directions:

Wash quinoa in a bowl, by rubbing vigorously between your hands. Discard water and repeat rinsing two more times.

On medium high fire, place a medium nonstick skillet.

Add cinnamon, vanilla extract, cherries and quinoa.

Bring to a boil and stir occasionally.

Once boiling, slow fire to a simmer, cover skillet and cook until all water is absorbed and quinoa is tender, around 15 minutes.

Turn off fire and let it stand covered for 10 minutes more.

Transfer to a serving bowl and if using honey, pour and mix.

Serve and enjoy.

Nutrition:

Calories: 386 Cal

Fat: 5.3 g

Carbs: 72.12 g

Protein: 13.0 g

Fiber: 7.7 g

66. Granola from Quinoa and Buckwheat

Preparation Time: 5 Minutes

Cooking Time: 45 Minutes

Servings 6

Ingredients: ½ cup old fashioned oats

½ cup dried unsweetened cranberries

1 cup cooked quinoa 1 cup buckwheat groats

¼ tsp ground ginger

¼ tsp ground cinnamon

1 tsp vanilla extract

1 tbsp liquid coconut oil

3 tbsp honey

Directions:

Grease a baking sheet and preheat oven to 325oF. In a large bowl, mix well oats, quinoa and buckwheat.

In a small bowl, stir well honey, coconut oil, vanilla, cinnamon, and ginger. Pour into bowl of oats and mix well. In an even layer, spread the mixture on baking sheet.

Pop into the oven and bake until grains begin to brown around 40 to 45 minutes. Remove from oven and stir in cranberries. Let it cool before serving or storing.

Nutrition: Calories: 146 Cal Fat: 4 g

Protein: 4 g Fiber: 3 g

67. Trout 'n Cannellini Tartine

Preparation Time: 10minutes

Cooking Time: 0 Minutes

Servings: 4

Ingredients: Dill sprigs – for garnish

4 large whole grain bread, toasted

1 tsp chopped fresh dill 2 tsp minced onion

1 stalk celery, finely chopped

½ 15-oz can cannellini beans

½ cup diced roasted red peppers

2 tbsp capers, rinsed and drained

¾ lb. smoked trout, flaked into bite-sized pieces

Pinch of sugar 1 tsp Dijon mustard

1 tbsp extra virgin olive oil

2 tbsp freshly squeezed lemon juice

Directions:

Mix sugar, mustard, olive oil and lemon juice in a big bowl. Add the rest of the ingredients except for toasted bread.

Toss to mix well.

Evenly divide fish mixture on top of bread slices and garnish with dill sprigs.

Serve and enjoy.

Nutrition: Calories: 253 Cal Fat: 9 g

Carbs: 17 g Protein: 25 g Fiber: 4 g

68. Brussels Sprouts 'n White Bean Medley

Prepration Time: 10 Minutes

Cooking Time: 20 Minutes

Servings: 4

Ingredients: Pepper to taste

6 garlic cloves, smashed, peeled, and minced

4 ½ cups Brussels sprouts, cleaned and sliced in half

3tbsp lemon juice

3 medium onions, peeled and sliced

3 cans white beans, drained and rinsed

1 tbsp olive oil 1 tsp salt

Directions:

Place a saucepan on medium high fire and heat for 2 minutes.

Add oil and heat for a minute.

Sauté garlic and onions for 3 minutes.

Stir in Brussels Sprouts and sauté for 5 minutes.

Stir in white beans and sauté for 5 minutes.

Season with pepper and salt.

Nutrition:

Calories 329 Fat 5g

Carbs 55g Protein 18g

Fiber 16g

69. Quinoa and Kidney Beans Pilaf

Preparation Time: 10 Minutes

Cooking Time: 40 Minutes

Servings: 4

Ingredients:

¼ teaspoon red pepper flakes

¼ teaspoon smoked paprika

½ teaspoon cumin

½ teaspoon sea salt

1 3/4 cups water

1 cup quinoa, uncooked

1 large clove garlic minced

1 small red bell pepper finely diced

1 small red onion finely diced

1 tablespoon tomato paste

1 15-ounce can kidney beans rinsed and drained

1 tsp olive oil

Directions:

Place a nonstick pot on medium high fire and heat oil for 2 minutes.

Stir in peppers and onion. Sauté for 5 minutes.

Add tomato paste, red pepper flakes, salt, paprika, cumin, and garlic. Sauté for 2 minutes.

Stir in quinoa and mix well. Sauté for 2 minutes.

Add water and beans. Mix well. Cover and simmer for 20 minutes or until liquid is fully absorbed.

Turn off fire and fluff quinoa. Let it sit for 5 minutes more while uncovered.

Serve and enjoy.

Nutrition:

Calories: 317 Cal Fat: 5 g

Carbs: 54 g Protein: 15 g Fiber: 10 g

Kidney Bean Salad with Vinaigrette

Preparation Time: 10 Minutes

Cooking Time: 10 Minutes

Servings: 4

Ingredients:

1 15-oz. can kidney beans, drained and rinsed

1/2 English cucumbers, chopped

1 Medium-sized heirloom tomato, chopped

1 bunch fresh cilantro, stems removed, chopped (about 1 1/4 cup)

1 red onion, chopped (about 1 cup)

Cilantro-Dijon Vinaigrette Ingredients:

1 large lime or lemon, juiced

3 tbsp extra virgin olive oil

1 tsp Dijon mustard

½ tsp fresh garlic paste, or finely chopped garlic

1 tsp sumac

Salt and pepper, to taste

Directions:

In a small bowl, whisk well all vinaigrette ingredients.

In a salad bowl, combine cilantro chopped veggies, and kidney beans.

Add vinaigrette to salad and toss well to mix.

For 30 minutes allow for flavors to mix and set in the fridge.

Mix and adjust seasoning if needed before serving.

Nutrition:

Calories: 250 Cal

Fat: 11 g

Carbs: 30 g

Protein: 10 g

Fiber: 8 g

Kidney Beans in Mexican Rice

Preparation Time: 10 Minutes

Cooking Time: 25 Minutes

Servings: 6

Ingredients:

2 tablespoons olive oil

2 cups julienned bell peppers

1 cup crushed tomatoes

1 cup corn kernels

2 tablespoons green chilies

1 tablespoon oregano

1 to 2 teaspoons chili powder to taste

3 cups cooked brown rice

Salt to taste

1/2 cup shredded purple cabbage

1 1/2 cups mixed veggies

1 1/2 teaspoons cumin

1/4 to 1/2 teaspoon liquid smoke to taste

1/4 cup minced onion

1 14.5 ounces can diced tomatoes

1 15.5 ounce can kidney beans

Directions

Place a large saucepan on medium high fire and heat for 2 minutes.

Add oil and heat for another 2 minutes. Stir in onions and sauté for 4 minutes.

Add cabbage and bell peppers, sauté for 3 minutes.

Stir in liquid smoke, chili powder, cumin, oregano, green chiles, corn, kidney beans, tomatoes, and mixed vegetables. Mix well.

Cover and cook for 9 minutes, mixing occasionally.

Stir in the cooked rice and lower fire to medium low. Mix rice well until colored red.

Adjust seasoning to taste, serve and enjoy one rice is heated through.

Nutrition:

Calories: 320 Cal

Fat: 8 g

Carbs: 55 g

Protein: 11 g

70. Green Hummus

Preparation Time: 10 Minutes

Cooking Time: 10 Minutes

Servings: 8

Ingredients:

¼ cup fresh lemon juice (about 1 large lemon's worth)

¼ cup roughly chopped, loosely packed fresh tarragon or basil - ¼ cup tahini

½ cup roughly chopped, loosely packed fresh parsley

½ teaspoon salt, more to taste

1 large garlic clove, roughly chopped

1 to 2 tablespoons water, optional

2 tablespoons olive oil, plus more for serving

2 to 3 tablespoons roughly chopped fresh chives or green onion

Garnish with extra olive oil and a sprinkling of chopped fresh herbs

One (15-ounce) can of chickpeas, also called garbanzo beans, drained and rinsed

Directions: Place al ingredients in a blender and puree until smooth and creamy. Transfer to a bowl and adjust seasoning if needed. Serve with pita chips.

Nutrition: Calories: 139 Cal Fat: 10 g

Carbs: 10 gProtein: 4 gFiber: 3 g

71. Parsley 'n Lemon Kidney Beans

Preparation Time: 10 Minutes

Cooking Time: 0

Servings: 6

Ingredients: 3 cloves garlic, pressed or minced

¼ cup lemon juice (about 1 ½ lemons)

¼ cup olive oil ¾ cup chopped fresh parsley

¾ teaspoon salt 1 small red onion, diced

1 can (15 ounces) chickpeas, rinsed and drained

1 medium cucumber, peeled, seeded and diced

2 cans (15 ounces each) red kidney beans, rinsed and drained

2 stalks celery, sliced in half or thirds lengthwise and chopped

2 tablespoons chopped fresh dill or mint

Small pinch red pepper flakes

Directions: Whisk well in a small bowl the pepper flakes, salt, garlic, and lemon juice until emulsified. In a serving bowl, combine the prepared kidney beans, chickpeas, onion, celery, cucumber, parsley and dill (or mint). Drizzle salad with the dressing and toss well to coat. Serve and enjoy.

Nutrition: Calories 345 Fat 11g

Carbs 47g Protein 16g Fiber 15g

72. Moroccan Salad

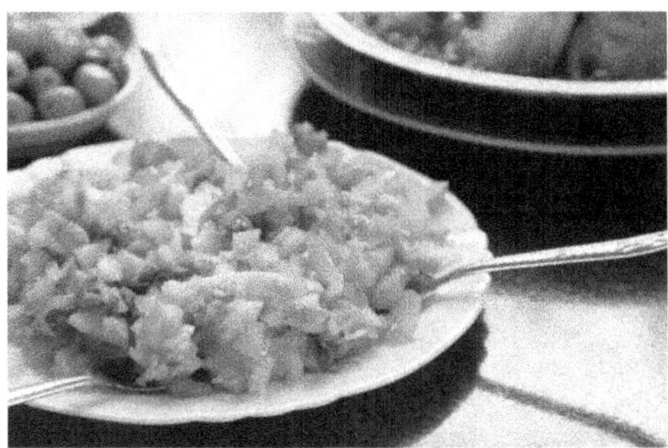

Preparation Time: 10 Minutes

Cooking Time: 0

Servings: 10

Ingredients:

¼ cup lemon juice

¼ teaspoon ground cinnamon

½ cup chopped fresh mint

½ cup extra-virgin olive oil

1 15-ounce can chickpeas, rinsed

1 cup finely diced carrot

1 small clove garlic, peeled and minced

1 teaspoon kosher salt, divided

1½ cups chopped fresh parsley

2 15-ounce cans dark red kidney beans, rinsed

2 tablespoons ground cumin

Directions:

In a salad bowl, whisk well lemon juice, cinnamon, olive oil, garlic, salt, parsley, and cumin.

Stir in remaining ingredients and toss well to coat in the dressing.

Serve and enjoy.

Nutrition:

Calories: 196 Cal Fat: 6 g

Carbs: 27 g Protein: 9 g

Fiber: 9 g

73. Blue Cheese 'n Pears on Grains Salad

Preparation Time: 10 minutes

Cooking Time: 40 minutes

Servings 4

Ingredients:

¼ cup thinly sliced scallions

½ cup millet, rinsed

½ cup quinoa, rinsed

1 ½ tsp olive oil

1 Bartlett pear, cored and diced

1/8 tsp ground black pepper

2 cloves garlic, minced

2 oz blue cheese

2 tbsp fresh lemon juice

2 tsp dried rosemary

4 4-oz boneless, skinless chicken breasts

6 oz baby spinach

olive oil cooking spray

Dressing Ingredients:

¼ cup fresh raspberries

1 tbsp pure maple syrup

1 tsp fresh thyme leaf

2 tbsp grainy mustard

6 tbsp balsamic vinegar

Directions:

Bring millet, quinoa, and 2 ¼ cups water on a small saucepan to a boil. Once boiling, slow fire to a simmer and stir once. Cover and cook until water is fully absorbed and grains are soft around 15 minutes. Turn off fire, fluff grains with a fork and set aside to cool a bit.

Arrange one oven rack to highest position and preheat broiler. Line a baking sheet with foil, and grease with cooking spray.

Whisk well pepper, oil, rosemary, lemon juice and garlic. Rub onto chicken.

Place chicken on prepared pan, pop into the broiler and broil until juices run clear and no longer pin inside around 12 minutes.

Meanwhile, make the dressing by combining all ingredients in a blender. Blend until smooth.

Remove chicken from oven, cool slightly before cutting into strips, against the grain.

To assemble, place grains in a large salad bowl. Add in dressing and spinach, toss to mix well.

Add scallions and pear, mix gently and evenly divide into four plates. Top each salad with cheese and chicken.

Serve and enjoy.

Nutrition:

Calories 415

Fat 9g

Carbs 53g

Protein 30g

Fiber 7g

74. Grains and Fruits

Preparation Time: 10 Minutes

Cooking Time: 20 Minutes

Servings: 6

Ingredients:

¼ tsp salt

¾ cup bulgur

¾ cup quick cooking brown rice

1 8-oz low fat vanilla yogurt

1 cup raisins

1 Granny Smith apple

1 orange

1 Red delicious apple

3 cups water

Directions:

On high fire, place a large pot and bring water to a boil.

Add bulgur and rice. Lower fire to a simmer and cook for ten minutes while covered.

Turn off fire, set aside for 2 minutes while covered.

In baking sheet, transfer and evenly spread grains to cool.

Meanwhile, peel oranges and cut into sections. Chop and core apples.

Once grains are cool, transfer to a large serving bowl along with fruits.

Add yogurt and mix well to coat.

Serve and enjoy.

Nutrition:

Calories: 118 Cal

Fat: 1 g

Carbs: 24 g

Protein: 4 g

Fiber: 4 g

75. Cherries and Quinoa

Preparation Time: 5 Minutes

Cooking Time: 10 Minutes

Servings1

Ingredients:

1 tsp honey – optional

¼ tsp ground cinnamon

½ tsp vanilla extract

½ cup dried unsweetened cherries

½ cup dry quinoa

1 cup water

Directions:

Wash quinoa in a bowl, by rubbing vigorously between your hands. Discard water and repeat rinsing two more times.

On medium high fire, place a medium nonstick skillet.

Add cinnamon, vanilla extract, cherries and quinoa.

Bring to a boil and stir occasionally.

Once boiling, slow fire to a simmer, cover skillet and cook until all water is absorbed and quinoa is tender, around 15 minutes.

Turn off fire and let it stand covered for 10 minutes more.

Transfer to a serving bowl and if using honey, pour and mix.

Serve and enjoy.

Nutrition:

Calories: 386 Cal

Fat: 5.3 g

Carbs: 72.12 g

Protein: 13 g

Fiber: 7.7 g

76. Granola from Quinoa and Buckwheat

Preparation Time: 5 Minutes

Cooking Time: 45 Minutes

Servings: 6

Ingredients: ½ cup old fashioned oats

½ cup dried unsweetened cranberries

1 cup cooked quinoa 1 cup buckwheat groats

¼ tsp ground ginger ¼ tsp ground cinnamon

1 tsp vanilla extract 1 tbsp liquid coconut oil

3 tbsp honey

Directions:

Grease a baking sheet and preheat oven to 325oF.

In a large bowl, mix well oats, quinoa and buckwheat.

In a small bowl, stir well honey, coconut oil, vanilla, cinnamon, and ginger. Pour into bowl of oats and mix well. In an even layer, spread the mixture on baking sheet.

Pop into the oven and bake until grains begin to brown around 40 to 45 minutes.

Remove from oven and stir in cranberries.

Let it cool before serving or storing.

Nutrition:

Calories: 146 Cal Fat: 4 g Carbs: 29 g

Protein: 4 g Fiber: 3 g

77. Trout 'n Cannellini Tartine

Preparation Time: 10 Minutes

Cooking Time: 0

Servings: 4

Ingredients: Dill sprigs – for garnish

4 large whole grain bread, toasted

1 tsp chopped fresh dill 2 tsp minced onion

1 stalk celery, finely chopped

½ 15-oz can cannellini beans

½ cup diced roasted red peppers

2 tbsp capers, rinsed and drained

¾ lb. smoked trout, flaked into bite-sized pieces

Pinch of sugar 1 tsp Dijon mustard

1 tbsp extra virgin olive oil

2 tbsp freshly squeezed lemon juice

Directions:

Mix sugar, mustard, olive oil and lemon juice in a big bowl. Add the rest of the ingredients except for toasted bread. Toss to mix well.

Evenly divide fish mixture on top of bread slices and garnish with dill sprigs. Serve and enjoy.

Nutrition:

Calories: 253 Cal Fat :9 g

Carbs 17 g Protein: 25 g Fiber: 4 g

78. Chipotle Style Rice

Preparation Time: 10 Minutes

Cooking Time: 17 Minutes

Servings: 10

Ingredients:

1 can vegetable broth

1 cup water

2 tablespoons canola oil

3 tablespoons juice of lime juice

2 cups long grain brown rice, rinsed

Zest of 1 lime

½ cup cilantro, chopped

½ teaspoon salt

Directions:

Place everything in the pot and give a good stir, except for lime juice, lime zest, and cilantro.

Cover and bring to a boil. Boil for 5 minutes.

Lower fire to a simmer and cook until liquid is fully absorbed, around 10 to 15 minutes.

Mix in remaining ingredients and let it stand for another 5 minutes.

Fluff the rice before serving.

Nutrition:

Calories: 166 Cal Fat: 4g Carbs: 30g

Protein: 3 g Fiber: 1 g

79. Rice & Currant Salad

Preparation Time: 10 Minutes

Cooking Time: 10 Minutes

Servings: 6

Ingredients:

1 cup brown basmati rice, uncooked

2 1/2 Tablespoons lemon juice

1 teaspoon grated orange zest

2 Tablespoons fresh orange juice

1/4 cup olive oil

1/2 teaspoon cinnamon

Salt and pepper to taste

4 chopped green onions

1/2 cup dried currants

3/4 cup shelled pistachios or almonds

1/4 cup chopped fresh parsley

Directions:

Place a nonstick pot on medium high fire and add rice. Toast rice until opaque and starts to smell, around 10 minutes.

Add 4 quarts of boiling water to pot and 2 tsp salt. Boil until tender, around 8 minutes uncovered.

Drain the rice and spread out on a lined cookie sheet to cool completely.

In a large salad bowl, whisk well the oil, juices and spices. Add salt and pepper to taste.

Add half of the green onions, half of parsley, currants, and nuts.

Toss with the cooled rice and let stand for at least 20 minutes.

If needed adjust seasoning with pepper and salt.

Garnish with remaining parsley and green onions.

Nutrition:

Calories: 365 Cal

Fat: 17 g

Carbs: 48 g

Protein: 8 g

Fiber: 5 g

80. Quinoa Pilaf

Preparation Time: 10 Minutes

Cooking Time: 20 Minutes

Servings 10

Ingredients:

2 tablespoons onion, chopped

1 tablespoon garlic, minced

2 tablespoons chopped celery

2 cups quinoa, rinsed

2 cups chicken broth

¾ teaspoon garlic powder

¼ teaspoon paprika

Salt and pepper to taste

1 tablespoon parsley, chopped

Directions:

Mix broth and quinoa in a saucepan.

Bring to a boil and reduce to a simmer.

Cover and cook for 10 minutes.

Stir in onions, garlic, celery, garlic powder, paprika, salt, and pepper. Cover and continue cooking for another 5 minutes or until liquid is fully absorbed.

Once liquid is fully absorbed, turn off fire and let stand for 5 min.

Fluff with a fork, then stir in parsley.

Nutrition:

Calories: 132 Cal

Fat: 2 g

Carbs: 23 g

Protein: 5 g

Fiber :3 g

Sauces and Staples Recipes

81. Honey-Mustard-Sesame Sauce

Preparations Time: 10 Minutes

Cooking Time: 0

Servings: 1

Ingredients:

Dijon mustard – ½ cup

Raw honey or maple syrup – ½ cup

Garlic – 1 clove, minced

Toasted sesame oil - 1 tsp.

Directions:

In a bowl, add everything and whisk to mix.

Store in the refrigerator.

Nutrition:

Calories: 67 Cal

Fat: 1 g

Carb: 14 g

Protein: 1 g

82. Ginger-Teriyaki Sauce

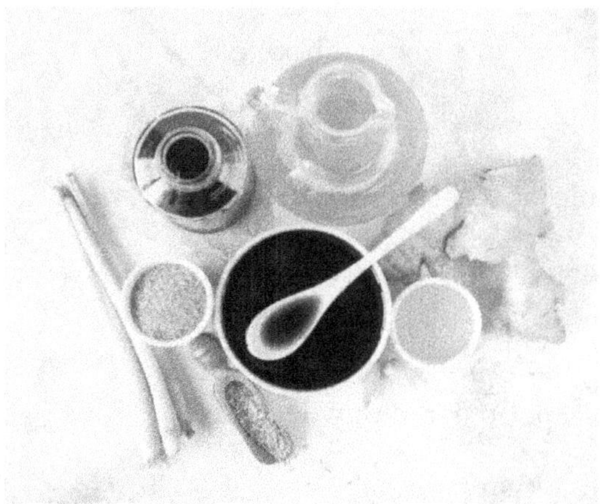

Preparation Time: 5 Minutes

Cooking Time: 0

Servings: 4

Ingredients Low sodium soy sauce – ¼ cup

No sugar added pineapple juice – ¼ cup

Raw honey – 2 Tbsps. Garlic powder – 1 tsp.

Grated fresh ginger - 1 Tbsp.

Arrowroot powder – 1 Tbsp.

Directions: Whisk everything in a bowl.

Store in the refrigerator.

Nutrition: Calories: 41 Cal Fat: 0 g

Carb: 10 g Protein: 1 g

83. Easy Garlicky Cherry Tomato Sauce

Preparation Time: 5 Minutes

Cooking Time: 25 Minutes

Servings: 4

Ingredients: ¼ cup extra virgin olive oil

¼ thinly sliced garlic cloves

2 pounds organic cherry tomatoes

½ teaspoon dried oregano

1 teaspoon coconut sugar

¼ cup chopped fresh basil 1 teaspoon salt

Directions:

Heat oil in a large saucepan over medium heat.

Sauté the garlic for a minute until fragrant.

Add in the cherry tomatoes and season with salt, oregano, coconut sugar, and fresh basil.

Allow to simmer for 25 minutes until the tomatoes are soft and becomes a thick sauce.

Place in containers and store in the fridge until ready to use.

Nutrition:

Calories: 198 Cal

Fat: 6 g

Carbs: 37 g Protein: 3 g

Fiber: 5 g

84. Avocado Cilantro Detox Dressing

Preparation Time: 5 Minutes

Cooking Time: 0

Servings 3

Ingredients:

5 tablespoons lemon juice, freshly squeezed

1 clove of garlic, chopped

1 avocado, pitted and flesh scooped out

1 bunch cilantro, chopped

¼ teaspoon salt

¼ cup water

Directions:

Place all ingredients in a food processor and pulse until well combined.

Pulse until creamy.

Place in a lidded container and store in the fridge until ready to use.

Use on salads and sandwiches.

Nutrition:

Calories 114 Cal

Fat: 10 g

Carbs: 8 g

Protein: 2 g Fiber: 5 g

85. Golden Turmeric Sauce

Preparation Time:10 Minutes

Cooking Time: 15 Minutes

Servings: 4

Ingredients: 2 tablespoons coconut oil

2-inch piece ginger, peeled and minced

2 cloves of garlic, minced

2 cups white sweet potato, cubed

2 tablespoons turmeric powder

½ teaspoon ginger powder

¼ teaspoon cinnamon powder

2 cups coconut milk 1 onion, chopped

Juice from 1 lemon, feshly squeezed

1 cup water 1 ½ teaspoon salt

Directions: Heat oil in a saucepan over medium flame. Sauté the onion, ginger, and garlic until fragrant. Add in the sweet potatoes, turmeric powder, ginger powder, and cinnamon powder. Pour in water and season with salt. Bring to a boil for 10 minutes. Once the potatoes are soft, place in a blender pulse until smooth. Return the mixture into the saucepan. Turn on the stove. Add in the coconut milk and lemon juice. Allow to simmer for 5 minutes. Store in lidded containers and put inside the fridge until ready to use.

Nutrition: Calories: 172 Cal Fat: 11 g

Carbs: 15 g Protein: 5 g Fiber: 3g

86. Creamy Turmeric Dressing

Preparation Time: 5 Minutes

Cooking Time: 0

Servings 6

Ingredients:

½ cup tahini

½ cup olive oil

2 tablespoons lemon juice

2 teaspoons honey

Salt to taste

a dash of black pepper

Directions:

Mix all ingredients in a bowl until the mixture becomes creamy and smooth.

Store in lidded containers.

Put in the fridge until ready to use.

Nutrition:

Calories 286

Fat 29g

Carbs 7g

Protein 4g

Fiber:2 g

87. Dijon Mustard Vinaigrette

Preparation Time: 5 Minutes

Cooking Time: 0

Servings: 6

Ingredients:

¾ cup olive oil

¼ cup apple cider vinegar

3 tablespoons Dijon mustard

2 shallots, quartered

1 garlic clove, chopped

A handful of parsley, chopped

Directions:

Place all ingredients in a food processor.

Pulse until smooth.

Place in containers and store in the fridge until ready to use.

Nutrition:

Calories: 252 Cal

Fat: 27 g

Carbs: 2 g

Protein: 0.6 g

Fiber: 0.7 g

88. Anti-Inflammatory Caesar Dressing

Preparation Time: 5 Minutes

Cooking Time: 0

Servings: 6

Ingredients:

½ cup cashew nuts, soaked in water then drained

1/3 cup fresh lemon juice

1 clove of garlic, minced

1 tablespoon Dijon mustard

1 tablespoon anchovy paste

2 tablespoon extra-virgin olive oil

½ cup plain Greek yogurt

Directions:

Place all ingredients in a food processor.

Pulse until a smooth paste is formed.

Place in containers and store in the fridge until ready to use.

Nutrition:

Calories: 96 Cal

Fat: 7 g

Carbs: 5 g

Protein: 4 g

Fiber: 0.5 g

89. Fresh Tomato Vinaigrette

Preparation Time: 5 Minutes

Cooking Time: 0

Servings 5

Ingredients:

1 fresh tomato, chopped

¾ cup olive oil

¼ cup apple cider vinegar

1 clove of garlic, chopped

½ teaspoon dried oregano

Salt and pepper to taste

Directions

Place all ingredients in a food processor.

Pulse until a smooth paste is formed.

Place in containers and store in the fridge until ready to use.

Nutrition:

Calories: 298 Cal

Fat: 32 g

Carbs: 2 g

Protein: 0.2 g

Fiber: 0.4 g

90. Ginger Sesame Sauce

Preparation Time: 5 Minutes

Cooking Time: 0

Servings: 6

Ingredients:

½ cup olive oil

¼ cup sesame oil

1/3 cup rice wine vinegar

1 tablespoon fresh ginger

1 tablespoon sesame seeds

Directions:

Place all ingredients in a food processor.

Pulse until a smooth paste is formed.

Place in containers and store in the fridge until ready to use.

Nutrition:

Calories: 250 Cal

Fat: 28 g

Carbs: 0.2 g

Protein: 0.3 g

Fiber: 0.1 g

91. Adobo Seasoning

Preparation Time: 10 Minutes

Cooking Time: 0

Servings: 40

Ingredients:

3 tablespoons garlic powder

1 teaspoon dried oregano, crushed

½ teaspoon ground cumin

2½ teaspoons salt

2 teaspoons freshly ground black pepper

Directions:

In a bowl, mix together all ingredients.

Store in an airtight jar.

Nutrition:

Calories: 3 Cal

Fat: 0 g

Carbs: 6 g

Fiber: 1 g

Protein: 1 g

92. Pumpkin Pie Spice

Preparation Time: 5 Minutes

Cooking Time: 0

Servings: 3

Ingredients:

1 teaspoon ground cinnamon

¼ teaspoon ground ginger

¼ teaspoon ground nutmeg

1/8 teaspoon ground cloves

Directions:

In a bowl, mix together all ingredients.

Store in an airtight jar.

Nutrition:

Calories: 6 Cal

Fat: 2g

Carbs: 4g

Fiber: 8g

Protein: 1g

93. Ginger-Garlic Paste

Preparation Time: 10 Minutes

Cooking Time: 0

Servings: 24

Ingredients:

4-ounce fresh ginger root, chopped

4-ounce garlic, chopped

1 tbsp olive oil

Directions:

In a food processor, add ginger and garlic and pulse till chopped finely.

While motor is running slowly, add oil and pulse till smooth.

Transfer the paste in an airtight jar and store in refrigerator.

Nutrition:

Calories: 24 Cal

Fat: 9g

Carbs: 6g

Fiber: 3g

Protein: 6g

94. Turmeric Paste

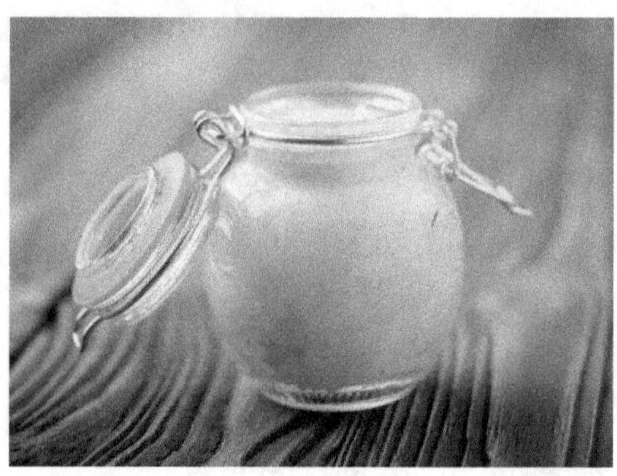

Preparation Time: 5 Minutes

Cooking Time: 0

Servings: 16

Ingredients:

1 cup raw honey

1 tablespoon coconut oil, softened

3 tablespoons ground turmeric

¼ teaspoon freshly ground black pepper

Directions:

In a sealable jar, add all ingredients and with a butter knife, mix well.

Refrigerate to store.

Nutrition:

Calories: 77 Cal

Fat: 1 g Carbs: 14 g

Fiber: 4 g

Protein: 2 g

95. Garlicky Harissa

Preparation Time: 15 Minutes

Cooking Time: 4 Minutes

Servings: 16

Ingredients:

8 dried New Mexico chiles, stemmed and seeded

8 dried guajillo chiles, stemmed and seeded

Boiling water, as required

½ teaspoon caraway seeds

¼ teaspoon cumin seeds

¼ teaspoon coriander seeds

1 teaspoon dried mint leaves

5 garlic cloves, chopped

3 tablespoons extra-virgin olive oil plus more, as needed

2 tablespoons fresh lemon juice

Salt, to taste

Directions:

In a bowl, add chiles and cover with boiling water.

Keep aside for about 20 minutes.

Meanwhile, heat a nonstick skillet on medium heat.

Add spice seeds and toast for about 4 minutes, swirling the skillet continuously.

In a grinder, add spice mixture and mint and pulse till powdered finely.

Drain the chiles completely.

In a food processor, add chiles, spice mixture and remaining ingredients and pulse till a smooth paste form.

Transfer the Harissa in a1-pint glass jar.

Add enough oil that will submerge the Harissa completely.

Nutrition:

Calories: 718 Cal

Fat: 0.9 g

Carbs: 11 g

Fiber: 5 g

Protein: 3 g

96. Sweet Potato Sauce

Preparation Time: 15 Minutes

Cooking Time: 16 Minutes

Servings: 24

Ingredients:

2 tablespoons coconut oil

1 onion, chopped

2 minced garlic cloves

1- 2-inchpiece fresh ginger, minced

2 cups white sweet potato, peeled and cubed

1 cup bone broth

2 tablespoons ground turmeric

½ tablespoon ground ginger

¼ teaspoon ground cinnamon

Salt, to taste

1- 13½-ouncecan coconut milk

2 tablespoons fresh lemon juice

Directions:

In a pan, melt coconut oil on medium heat.

Add onion and sauté for about 5minutes.

Add garlic and ginger and sauté for about 1 minute.

Add sweet potato, broth and spices and bring to a boil.

Reduce the heat to low and simmer, covered for about 10 minutes.

Remove from heat and keep aside to cool for about 5 minutes.

In a blender, add sweet potato mixture and remaining ingredients and pulse till smooth.

Nutrition:

Calories: 76 Cal

Fat: 1 g

Carb: 11 g

Protein: 2 g

97. Tomato Sauce- Ketchup

Preparation Time: 15 Minutes

Cooking Time: 2 Hours 22 Minutes

Servings: 4-6

Ingredients:

1 tbsp olive oil

1 yellow onion, chopped

1- 1-inchpiece fresh ginger, minced

4 garlic cloves, minced

3 tablespoons tomato paste

1 teaspoon ground mustard

½ teaspoon cayenne pepper

½ teaspoon paprika

¼ teaspoon ground coriander

1/8 teaspoon ground cloves

2 bay leaves

1- 28-ouncecan diced tomatoes

¼ cup coconut crystals

½ cup coconut vinegar

Salt, to taste

Directions:

In a pan, heat oil on medium-high heat.

Add onion and sauté for about 5 minutes.

Add ginger and garlic and sauté for about 1 minute.

Stir in tomato paste and spices and sauté for about 1 minute.

Stir in remaining ingredients and reduce the heat to medium.

Simmer, stirring occasionally for about 15 minutes.

Remove from heat and keep aside to cool slightly.

In a blender, add tomato mixture and pulse till smooth.

Return the mixture into pan on low heat.

Simmer, stirring occasionally for about 2 hours.

Nutrition:

Calories: 97 Cal

Fat: 2 g

Carb: 24 g

Protein: 1 g

98. Scallion Sauce

Preparation Time: 15 Minutes

Cooking Time: 5 Minutes

Servings: 4-6

Ingredients:

2 cups scallions, chopped finely

1/3 cup fresh ginger, minced

1 teaspoon Aleppo pepper

Salt, to taste

¼ cup coconut oil

2 tablespoons extra-virgin olive oil

Directions:

In a large glass bowl, mix together all ingredients except both oils.

In a small pan, melt coconut oil for about 3-5 minutes.

Place the hot oil over scallion mixture evenly.

After 1-2 minutes, add olive oil and stir to combine well.

Nutrition:

Calories: 88 Cal

Fat: 0.7 g

Carb: 13 g

Protein: 3 g

99. Beet Sauce

Preparation Time: 15 Minutes

Cooking Time: 1 Hour

Servings: 6

Ingredients: 2 garlic cloves, chopped

2-pound beets, peeled and cubed

1 tablespoon coconut oil, melted

2 tablespoons fresh lemon juice

1 tablespoon apple cider vinegar

¼ cup water Salt, to taste

1/3 cup extra-virgin olive oil

Directions:

Preheat the oven to 400 degrees F.

Coat the beet cubes with coconut oil evenly.

Place the beet cubes in a baking dish.

Bake for about 1 hour, stirring after every 20 minutes.

Remove from oven and keep aside to cool for about 10 minutes.

In a food processor, add beets and remaining ingredients except olive oil and pulse till well combined.

While motor is running slowly, add oil pulsing continuously till smooth.

Nutrition: Calories: 57 Cal Fat: 19 g

Carb:27 g Protein: 7 g

100.   Eggplant Sauce- Baba Ghanoush

Preparation Time: 15 Minutes

Cooking Time: 35 Minutes

Servings: 8

Ingredients: 2 large eggplants

2 garlic cloves, chopped 2 tablespoons tahini

2 tablespoons fresh lemon juice

3 teaspoons extra-virgin olive oil

1 teaspoon ground cumin

Salt and freshly ground black pepper, to taste

Olive oil, for drizzling

Chopped fresh parsley leaves, for garnishing

Directions:

Preheat the oven to 400 degrees F. Grease a baking dish. Place the eggplants in prepared baking dish.

Bake for about 35 minutes.

Remove from oven and immediately, place in bowl of cold water to cool slightly.

Peel off the skin of eggplants.

In a food processor, add eggplants and remaining ingredients except olive oil and parsley and pulse till smooth.

Refrigerate to chill before.

While, drizzle with olive oil and garnish with parsley.

Vegetarian and Vegan Recipes

101. Nutty and Fruity Garden Salad

Preparation time: 10 minutes

Cooking time: 0 minutes

Servings: 2

Ingredients: 6 cups baby spinach

½ cup chopped walnuts, toasted

1 ripe red pear, sliced

1 ripe persimmon, sliced

1 teaspoon garlic minced   1 shallot, minced

1 tablespoon extra-virgin olive oil

2 tablespoons fresh lemon juice

1 teaspoon whole grain mustard

Directions:

Mix well garlic, shallot, oil, lemon juice and mustard in a large salad bowl.

Add spinach, pear and persimmon. Toss to coat well.

To serve, garnish with chopped pecans.

Nutrition:

Calories 332 Fat 21g Carbs 37g

Protein 7g Fiber 9g

102. Creamy Cauliflower-Broccoli Soup

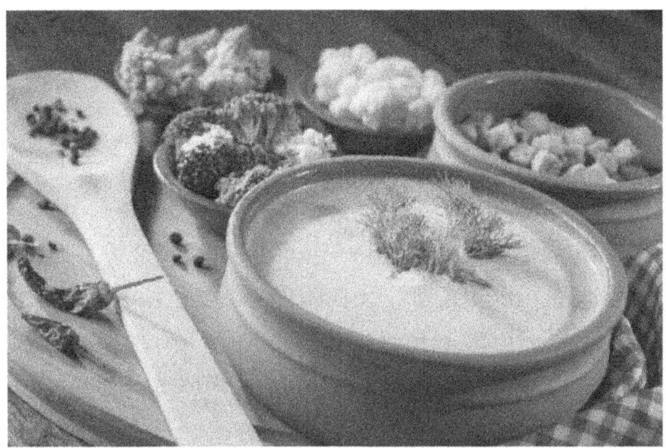

Preparation time: 15 minutes

Cooking time: 15 minutes

Servings: 6

Ingredients:

Pepper and salt to taste

4 cups chicken broth

1 teaspoon dried basil

1 teaspoon dried oregano

½ cup onion, roughly chopped

2 cups carrots, cubed

3 cups cauliflower florets

2 cups broccoli florets

Directrions:

In a large soup pot, bring to a boil chicken broth, basil, oregano and onions. Once boiling, lower fire to a simmer.

Meanwhile, dice cauliflower and broccoli florets. And add to pot. Add carrots, cover and simmer for 10 minutes. Season with pepper and salt to taste.

Turn off fire and allow soup to cool.

Place veggies into a blender while ensuring that liquid is reserved. Puree veggies along with 1 cup of reserved liquid. If you want a thick soup, then 1 cup liquid is enough. If you desire a less thick soup, add more reserved liquid until desired consistency is reached.

Return pureed soup to empty pot and simmer until heated through. Adjust seasoning if needed before serving.

Nutrition:

Calories 39

Fat 0.3g

Carbs 8g

Protein 2g

Fiber 3g

103.   Nutty and Fruity Amaranth Porridge

Preparation time: 10 minutes

Cooking time: 30 minutes

Servings: 2

Ingredients:

1 medium pear, chopped

½ cup blueberries

1 tsp cinnamon

1 tbsp raw honey

¼ cup pumpkin seeds

2 cups filtered water

2/3 cups whole-grain amaranth

Directions:

In a nonstick pan with cover, boil water and amaranth. Slow fire to a simmer and continue cooking until liquid is absorbed completely, around 25-30 minutes.

Turn off fire.

Mix in cinnamon, honey and pumpkin seeds. Mix well.

Pour equally into two bowls.

Garnish with pear and blueberries.

Serve and enjoy.

Nutrition: Calories 416 Fat 12g

Carbs 68g Protein 14g Fiber 7g

104. Korean Barbecue Tofu

Preparation time: 10 minutes

Cooking time: 15 minutes

Servings: 3

Ingredients: 1 tbsp olive oil

2 tsp onion powder

4 garlic cloves, minced   2 tsp dry mustard

3 tbsp brown sugar   ½ cup soy sauce

1 ½ lbs. firm tofu, sliced to ¼-inch cubes

Directions

In a re-sealable bag, mix all ingredients except for tofu and oil. Mix well until sugar is dissolved.

Add sliced tofu and slowly turn bag to mmix. Seal bag and place flatly inside the ref for an hour.

After an hour, turn bag to the other side and marinate for another hour.

To cook, in a nonstick fry pan, heat oil on medium high fire. Add tofu and stir fry until sides are browned.

Serve and enjoy.

Nutrition: Calories 437

Fat 25g Carbs 23g

Protein 40g

Fiber 6g

105. Fruit Bowl with Yogurt Topping

Preparation time: 15 minutes

Cooking time: 0 minutes

Servings: 6

Ingredients: ¼ cup golden brown sugar

2/3 cup minced fresh ginger

1 16-oz Greek yogurt

¼ tsp ground cinnamon   2 tbsp honey

½ cup dried cranberries

3 navel oranges   2 large tangerines

1 pink grapefruit, peeled

Directions:

Into sections, break tangerines and grapefruit.

Slice tangerine sections in half and grapefruit sections into thirds. Place all sliced fruits and its juices in a large bowl.

Peel oranges, remove pith, slice into ¼-inch thick rounds and then cut into quarters. Transfer to bowl of fruit along with juices. In bowl, add cinnamon, honey and ¼ cup of cranberries. Place in the ref for an hour. In a medium bowl mix ginger and yogurt. Place on top of fruit bowl, drizzle with remaining cranberries and brown sugar.

Serve and enjoy.

Nutrition: Calories 171 Fat 1g

Carbs 35g Protein 9g Fiber 3g

106. Mushroom, Spinach and Turmeric Frittata

Preparation time: 10 minutes

Cooking time: 40 minutes

Servings: 6

Ingredients:

½ tsp pepper

½ tsp salt

1 tsp turmeric

5-oz firm tofu

4 large eggs

6 large egg whites

¼ cup water

1 lb. fresh spinach

6 cloves freshly chopped garlic

1 large onion, chopped

1 lb. button mushrooms, sliced

Directions:

Grease a 10-inch nonstick and oven proof skillet and preheat oven to 350oF.

Place skillet on medium high fire and add mushrooms. Cook until golden brown.

Add onions, cook for 3 minutes or until onions are tender.

Add garlic, sauté for 30 seconds.

Add water and spinach, cook while covered until spinach is wilted, around 2 minutes.

Remove lid and continue cooking until water is fully evaporated.

In a blender, puree pepper, salt, turmeric, tofu, eggs and egg whites until smooth. Pour into skillet once liquid is fully evaporated.

Pop skillet into oven and bake until the center is set around 25-30 minutes.

Remove skillet from oven and let it stand for ten minutes before inverting and transferring to a serving plate.

Cut into 6 equal wedges, serve and enjoy.

Nutrition:

Calories 358

Fat 6g

Carbs 65g

Protein 21g

Fiber 12g

107.   Roasted Root Vegetables

Preparation time: 10 minutes

Cooking time: 1 hour and 30 minutes

Servings: 6

Ingredients:

2 tbsp olive oil

1 head garlic, cloves separated and peeled

1 large turnip, peeled and cut into ½-inch pieces

1 medium sized red onion, cut into ½-inch pieces

1 ½ lbs. beets, trimmed but not peeled, scrubbed and cut into ½-inch pieces

1 ½ lbs. Yukon gold potatoes, unpeeled, cut into ½-inch pieces

2 ½ lbs. butternut squash, peeled, seeded, cut into ½-inch pieces

Directions:

Grease 2 rimmed and large baking sheets. Preheat oven to 425oF.

In a large bowl, mix all ingredients thoroughly.

Into the two baking sheets, evenly divide the root vegetables, spread in one layer.

Season generously with pepper and salt.

Pop into the oven and roast for 1 hour and 15 minute or until golden brown and tender.

Remove from oven and let it cool for at least 15 minutes before serving.

Nutrition:

Calories 278 Fat 5g

Carbs 57g Protein 6g Fiber 10g

108.   Tropical Fruit Parfait

Preparation time: 10 minutes

Cooking time: 10 minutes

Servings: 1

Ingredients:

1 tbsp toasted sliced almonds

¼ cup plain soy yogurt

½ cup of fruit combination cut into ½-inch cubes (pineapple, mango and kiwi)

Instructions:

Prepare fresh fruit by peeling and slicing into ½-inch cubes.

Place cubed fruit in a bowl and top with a dollop of soy yogurt.

Garnish with sliced almonds and if desired, refrigerate for an hour before serving.

Nutrition:

Calories 119 Fat 2g

Carbs 25g Protein 2g Fiber 1g

109. Cinnamon Chips with Avocado-Strawberry Salsa

Preparation time: 10 minutes

Cooking time: 10 minutes

Servings: 6

Ingredients:

3/8 tsp salt

2 tsp fresh lime juice

1 tsp minced seeded jalapeno pepper

2 tbsp minced fresh cilantro

1 cup finely chopped strawberries

1 ½ cups finely chopped, peeled and ripe avocado

½ tsp ground cinnamon

2 tsp sugar

6 6-inch brown rice tortillas

2 tsp olive oil

Directions:

Preheat oven to 350oF.

Prepare the cinnamon chips by brushing olive oil all over the brown rice tortilla.

In a small bowl, mix together cinnamon and sugar.

Sprinkle cinnamon-sugar mixture evenly all over each of the brown rice tortilla.

Cut up each tortilla into 12 wedges, evenly and place on a baking sheet. If needed you can bake tortilla in two batches.

Pop the tortillas into the oven and bake until crisped, around 10 minutes. Remove from oven and keep warm.

Meanwhile, prepare salsa by mixing the remaining ingredients in a medium bowl. Stir to mix well.

To enjoy, dip crisped tortillas into bowl of salsa and eat or, you can spread the fruity salsa all over one tortilla chip and enjoy.

Nutrition:

Calories 213

Fat 11g

Carbs 25g

Protein 5g

Fiber 7g

110. Stir Fried Brussels Sprouts and Carrots

Preparation time: 10 minutes

Cooking time: 15 minutes

Servings: 6

Ingredients:

1 tbsp cider vinegar

1/3 cup water

1 lb. Brussels sprouts, halved lengthwise

1 lb. carrots cut diagonally into ½-inch thick lengths

3 tbsp olive oil, divided

2 tbsp chopped shallot

½ tsp pepper

¾ tsp salt

Directions:

On medium high fire, place a nonstick medium fry pan and heat 2 tbsp oil.

Ass shallots and cook until softened, around one to two minutes while occasionally stirring.

Add pepper salt, Brussels sprouts and carrots. Stir fry until vegetables starts to brown on the edges, around 3 to 4 minutes.

Add water, cook and cover.

After 5 to 8 minutes, or when veggies are already soft, add remaining butter.

If needed season with more pepper and salt to taste.

Turn off fire, transfer to a platter, serve and enjoy.

Nutrition:

Calories 98 Fat 4g Carbs 14g

Protein 3 Fiber 5g

111. Curried Veggies and Poached Eggs

Preparation time: 10 minutes

Cooking time: 50 minutes

Servings: 4

Ingredients: 4 large eggs

½ tsp white vinegar

1/8 tsp crushed red pepper – optional

1 cup water

1 14-oz can chickpeas, drained

2 medium zucchinis, diced

½ lb. sliced button mushrooms

1 tbsp yellow curry powder

2 cloves garlic, minced

1 large onion, chopped

2 tsp extra virgin olive oil

Directions:

On medium high fire, place a large saucepan and heat oil.

Sauté onions until tender around four to five minutes.

Add garlic and continue sautéing for another half minute.

Add curry powder, stir and cook until fragrant around one to two minutes.

Add mushrooms, mix, cover and cook for 5 to 8 minutes or until mushrooms are tender and have released their liquid.

Add red pepper if using, water, chickpeas and zucchini. Mix well to combine and bring to a boil.

Once boiling, reduce fire to a simmer, cover and cook until zucchini is tender around 15 to 20 minutes of simmering.

Meanwhile, in a small pot filled with 3-inches deep of water, bring to a boil on high fire.

Once boiling, reduce fire to a simmer and add vinegar.

Slowly add one egg, slipping it gently into the water. Allow to simmer until egg is cooked, around 3 to 5 minutes.

Remove egg with a slotted spoon and transfer to a plate, one plate one egg.

Repeat the process with remaining eggs.

Once the veggies are done cooking, divide evenly into 4 servings and place one serving per plate of egg.

Serve and enjoy.

Nutrition: Calories 254 Fat 9g Carbs 30g

Protein 16g Fiber 9g

112.   Braised Kale

Preparation Time: 10minutes

Cooking Time: 15 minutes

Servings 3

Ingredients: 2 to 3 tbsp water

1 tbsp coconut oil ½ sliced red pepper

2 stalk celery (sliced to ¼-inch thick)

5 cups of chopped kale

Directions:

Heat a pan over medium heat.   Add coconut oil and sauté the celery for at least five minutes. Add the kale and red pepper.

Add a tablespoon of water.

Let the vegetables wilt for a few minutes. Add a tablespoon of water if the kale starts to stick to the pan.   Serve warm.

Nutrition: Calories 61 Fat 5g

Carbs 3g Protein 1g

Fiber 1g,

113. Braised Leeks, Cauliflower and Artichoke Hearts

Preparation Time: 10 minutes

Cooking Time: 10 minutes

Servings 4

Ingredients:

2 tbsp coconut oil

2 garlic cloves, chopped

1 ½ cup artichoke hearts

1 ½ cups chopped leeks

1 ½ cups cauliflower flowerets

Directions:

Heat oil in a skillet over medium high heat.

Add the garlic and sauté for one minute. Add the vegetables and stir constantly until the vegetables are cooked.

Serve with roasted chicken, fish or pork.

Nutrition:

Calories 111

Fat 7g

Carbs 12g

Protein 3g

Fiber 4g

114. Celery Root Hash Browns

Preparation Time: 10 minutes

Cooking Time: 10 minutes

Servings 4

Ingredients:

4 tbsp coconut oil

½ tsp sea salt

2 to 3 medium celery roots

Directions:

Scrub the celery root clean and peel it using a vegetable peeler.

Grate the celery root in a food processor or a manual grater.

In a skillet, add oil and heat it over medium heat.

Place the grated celery root on the skillet and sprinkle with salt.

Let it cook for 10 minutes on each side or until the grated celery turns brown.

Serve warm.

Nutrition:

Calories 160

Fat 14g Fat 3g

Carbs 10g

Protein 1.5g Fiber 3g

115. Zucchini Pasta with Avocado Sauce

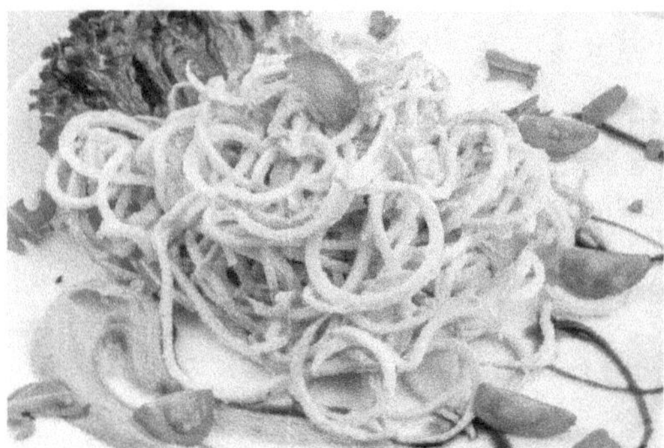

Preparations Time: 10 minutes

Cooking Time: 10 minutes

Servings 1

Ingredients: A squeeze of lemon juice

Salt and pepper to taste 1 tbsp coconut milk

½ ripe avocado 2 tbsp olive oil

1 medium zucchini cut into noodles

Directions:

Heat the oil in a skillet over medium heat and add the zucchini noodles. Sauté for three minutes or until the noodles have softened.

While the zucchini is cooking, mash the avocado together with the coconut milk, lemon juice and salt and pepper. Add the sauce to the zucchini noodles and sauté. Serve warm.

Nutrition: Calories 471 Fat 43g

Carbs 23g Protein 6g Fiber 9g

Blueberry Chia Pudding

Preparations Time: 10 minutes

Cooking Time: 10 minutes

Servings 2

Ingredients:

½ cup chia seeds

½ of frozen banana

5 dates (soaked in water)

2/3 cup almond milk

2 cups frozen blueberries

Directions:

Combine the milk, blueberries, dates and bananas in a blender. Process until the mixture becomes smooth.

Transfer the blueberry to a bowl and add the chia seeds.

Refrigerate for 30 minutes or overnight if necessary, until the chia seeds forms mucilage.

Serve with your favorite fruit or nut toppings.

Nutrition:

Calories 343

Fat 13g

Carbs 55g

Protein 9g

Fiber 16g,

Collard Green Wrap

Preparation Time: 10 minutes

Cooking Time: 0 minutes

Servings 4

Ingredients:

½ block feta, cut into 4 (1-inch thick) strips (4-oz)

½ cup purple onion, diced

½ medium red bell pepper, julienned

1 medium cucumber, julienned

4 large cherry tomatoes, halved

4 large collard green leaves, washed

8 whole kalamata olives, halved

Sauce Ingredients:

1 cup low-fat plain Greek yogurt

1 tablespoon white vinegar

1 teaspoon garlic powder

2 tablespoons minced fresh dill

2 tablespoons olive oil

2.5-ounces cucumber, seeded and grated (¼-whole)

Salt and pepper to taste

Directions:

Make the sauce first: make sure to squeeze out all the excess liquid from the cucumber after grating. In a small bowl, mix all sauce ingredients thoroughly and refrigerate.

Prepare and slice all wrap ingredients.

On a flat surface, spread one collard green leaf. Spread 2 tablespoons of Tzatziki sauce on middle of the leaf.

Layer ¼ of each of the tomatoes, feta, olives, onion, pepper, and cucumber. Place them on the center of the leaf, like piling them high instead of spreading them.

Fold the leaf like you would a burrito. Repeat process for remaining ingredients.

Serve and enjoy.

Nutrition:

Calories 463

Fat 31g

Carbs 31g

Protein 20g

Fiber 7g

116. Zucchini Garlic Fries

Preparation Time: 10 minutes

Cooking Time: 20 minutes

Servings 6

Ingredients:

¼ teaspoon garlic powder

½ cup almond flour

2 large egg whites, beaten

3 medium zucchinis, sliced into fry sticks

Salt and pepper to taste

Directions:

Preheat oven to 400oF.

Mix all ingredients in a bowl until the zucchini fries are well coated.

Place fries on cookie sheet and spread evenly.

Put in oven and cook for 20 minutes.

Halfway through cooking time, stir fries.

Nutrition:

Calories 11

Fat 0.1g,

Carbs 1g

Protein1.5 g

Fiber 0.5g

117. Mashed Cauliflower

Preparation Time: 10 minutes

Cooking Time: 10 minutes

Servings 3

Ingredients:

1 cauliflower head

1 tablespoon olive oil

½ tsp salt

¼ tsp dill

Pepper to taste

2 tbsp low fat milk

Directions:

Bring a small pot of water to a boil.

Chop cauliflower in florets.

Add florets to boiling water and boil uncovered for 5 minutes. Turn off fire and let it sit for 5 minutes more.

In a blender, add all ingredients except for cauliflower and blend to mix well.

Drain cauliflower well and add into blender. Puree until smooth and creamy.

Serve and enjoy.

Nutrition: Calories 78

Fat 5g Carbs 6g

Protein 2g Fiber 2g

118.   Stir-Fried Eggplant

Preparation Time: 10 minutes

Cooking Time: 10 minutes

Servings 2

Ingredients: 1 tablespoon coconut oil

2 eggplants, sliced into 3-inch in length

4 cloves of garlic, minced

1 onion, chopped 1 teaspoon ginger, grated

1 teaspoon lemon juice, freshly squeezed

½ tsp salt

½ tsp pepper

Directions:

Heat oil in a nonstick saucepan.

Pan-fry the eggplants for 2 minutes on all sides.

Add the garlic and onions until fragrant, around 3 minutes.

Stir in the ginger, salt, pepper, and lemon juice.

Add a ½ cup of water and bring to a simmer. Cook until eggplant is tender.

Nutrition:

Calories 232

Fat 8g Carbs 41g

Protein 7g Fiber 18g

119.   Sautéed Garlic Mushrooms

Preparation Time: 10 minutes

Cooking Time: 10 minutes

Servings 4

Ingredients:

1 tablespoon olive oil

3 cloves of garlic, minced

16 ounces fresh brown mushrooms, sliced

7 ounces fresh shiitake mushrooms, sliced

½ tsp salt

½ tsp pepper or more to taste

Directions:

Place a nonstick saucepan on medium high fire and heat pan for a minute.

Add oil and heat for 2 minutes.

Stir in garlic and sauté for a minute.

Add remaining ingredients and stir fry until soft and tender, around 5 minutes.

Turn off fire, let mushrooms rest while pan is covered for 5 minutes.

Serve and enjoy.

Nutrition:

Calories 95 Fat 4g Carbs 14g Protein 3g,

Fiber 4g

120. Stir Fried Asparagus and Bell Pepper

Preparation Time: 10 minutes

Cooking Time: 10 minutes

Servings 6

Ingredients:

1 tablespoon olive oil

4 cloves of garlic, minced

1-pound fresh asparagus spears, trimmed

2 large red bell peppers, seeded and julienned

½ teaspoon thyme

5 tablespoons water

½ tsp salt

½ tsp pepper or more to taste

Directions:

Place a nonstick saucepan on high fire and heat pan for a minute.

Add oil and heat for 2 minutes.

Stir in garlic and sauté for a minute.

Add remaining ingredients and stir fry until soft and tender, around 6 minutes.

Turn off fire, let veggies rest while pan is covered for 5 minutes.

Nutrition:

Calories 45

Fat 2g

Carbs 5g, Net

Protein 2g

Fiber 2g

Dessert Recipes

121. A Skillet Full of Granola

Preparation Time: 7 Minutes

Cooking Time: 12 Minutes

Servings: 3

Ingredients 6 pieces of pitted Mejdool dates

¼ cup of boiling water

1 tablespoon of coconut oil (melted)

1 tablespoon of cinnamon

¼ teaspoon of sea salt 2 cups of rolled oats

1 cup of raw nuts

Directions:

Take a food processor and add water, dates, cinnamon, oil, salt and puree the whole mixture until smooth Transfer it to a large sized bowl and stir in your oats, seeds and nuts Take a 12 inch skillet and place it over medium heat Add the mixture and cook it for about 12 minutes, making sure to keep stirring it regularly Let it cool and serve!

Nutrition:

Calories: 132 Cal Fat: 6 g

Carbs: 18 g Protein: 2.8 g

122. Feisty Chia and Oatmeal Cookies

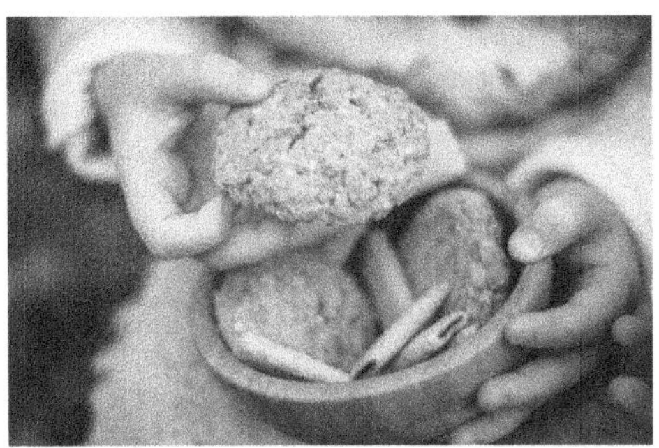

Preparation Time: 15 Minutes

Cooking Time: 10 Minutes

Servings: 4

Ingredients:

2 cups of rolled oatmeal

1 cup of brown sugar

2/3 cup of whole wheat flour

2 tablespoon of chia seeds

1 teaspoon of cinnamon, ground

1 teaspoon of baking soda

½ a teaspoon of baking powder

½ a teaspoon of salt

2/3 cup of applesauce

3 tablespoon of coconut oil

1 cup of dried cranberries

½ a cup of chocolate chips

¼ cup of unsweetened coconut, shredded

Directions:

Pre-heat your oven to 350-degree Fahrenheit

Take a bowl and add oats, flour, sugar, chia seeds, baking soda, cinnamon, baking powder and salt

Line up a baking sheet with parchment paper

Mix well

Stir in your applesauce alongside coconut oil into the oat mix and keep mixing until you have a even dough

Fold in chocolate chips (if using), cranberries and coconut

Spoon up the dough into your baking sheet

Bake for 10-15 minutes and enjoy!

Nutrition:

Calories: 262 Cal

Fats: 8 g

Carbs:47 g

Protein:3.4 g

123. Traditional Orange (Vegan) Cake

Preparation Time: 15 Minutes

Cooking Time: 30 Minutes

Servings: 4

Ingredients   1 large sized orange, peeled

1 and a ½ cups of all-purpose flour

1 cup of white sugar   ½ a cup of vegetable oil

1 and a ½ teaspoon of baking soda

¼ teaspoon of salt

Directions:

Pre-heat your oven to 375 degree Fahrenheit

Take an 8x8 inch baking pan and grease it up well

Take a blender and blend in orange, making sure to get at least 1 cup of orange juice

Take a bowl and whisk in orange juice, vegetable oil, sugar, baking soda, and salt

Mix well and pour the prepared batter into your pan

Bake for about 30 minutes until a toothpick comes out clean from the center

Enjoy!

Nutrition: Calories: 157 Cal

Fats: 7 g Carbs:22 g Protein:1.3 g

124.   Ravishing Choco-Nut Banana Bites

Preparation Time: 10 Minutes

Cooking Time: 0

Servings: 4

Ingredients:

4 teaspoons of cocoa powder

4 teaspoons of toasted unsweetened coconut

2 sliced of small bananas

Directions:

Take two individual plates and place the cocoa and coconut on those plates (individually)

Roll up the banana slices in the cocoa first and shake off any excess

Then dip them in the coconut

Serve!

Nutrition:

Protein: 1 g

Carbs: 13 g

Fats: 1 g

Calories: 60 Cal

125.   Very Cool And "Offbeat" Melon Soup

Preparation Time: 15 Minutes

Cooking Time: 0

Servings: 4

Ingredients

4 cups of casaba melon, cubed and seeded

¾ cup of coconut milk

Juice of 2 lime

1 tablespoon ginger, grated

1 pinch of salt

Directions:

Add the coconut milk, casaba melon, lime juice, salt and ginger to your food processor

Process it for about 1-2 minutes until the mixture has a soup like texture

Enjoy!

Nutrition:

Calories: 134 Cal

Fats: 9 g

Carbs:13 g

Protein:2 g

126. Fantastic Almond "Vegan" Butter Balls

Preparation Time: 10 Minutes

Cooking Time: 0

Servings: 4

Ingredients

12 dates, pitted and diced

1/3 cup of unsweetened shredded coconut

2 and a ½ tablespoon of almond butter

Directions:

Take a bowl and add dates, almond butter and coconut

Mix well

Use the mixture to form small balls

Store them in your fridge and chill them

Enjoy!

Nutrition:

Calories: 62 Cal

Fats: 3 g

Carbs:8 g

Protein:1 g

127. Fancy Coconut Date Bars For A Lovely Evening

Preparation Time: 10 Minutes

Cooking Time: 30 Minutes

Servings: 4

Ingredients:

1/3 cup of slivered almonds

½ a cup coconut, flaked

10 dates, pitted

¼ cup of cashews

1 teaspoon of coconut oil

Directions:

Take a food processor and ad the almonds, blend them

Add dates and pulse until mixed well

Add coconut oil and cashews until the mix is thick and sticks together

Transfer the mixture to a wax paper and form nice squares

Fold up the sides of the waxed-on top

Chill for at least 30 minutes and serve

Enjoy!

Nutrition: Calories: 154 Cal

Fats: 0 g Carbs: 39 g

Protein: 0.1 g

128. Vegan Coconut Whipped Cream

Preparation Time: 8 Hours 10 Minutes

Cook Time: 0

Servings: 6

Ingredients: 2 tablespoons of white sugar

1 can of unsweetened coconut milk

1 teaspoon of pure vanilla extract

Directions:

Place the can of coconut in your fridge and allow it to chill for 8 hours

Make sure to chill a metal bowl and beats in your fridge for about 1 hour prior to preparing the whip

Open up your coconut milk can and scoop out the coconut cream solids into your metal bowl Keep the liquids for later use

Beat the cream using a mixer on medium speed

Set the speed on HIGH and beat for 7-8 minutes until stiff peaks form

Add sugar, vanilla extract to the coconut cream and beat for 1 minute more Give it a taste and add more sugar if needed

Enjoy with cakes of muffins!

Nutrition:

Calories: 11 Cal Fats: 0 g

Carbs: 2.4 g Protein: 0 g

129. Thar She' Salts Peanut Butter Cookies

Preparation Time: 15 Minutes

Cooking Time: 0

Servings: 9

Ingredients

1 cup of raw almonds

½ a cup of peanut butter (creamy and unsalted)

1 cup of pitted Mejdool dates

1 and a ¼ teaspoon of vanilla extract

Sea salt as needed

Directions:

Take a food processor and add almonds, peanut butter, vanilla, dates and blend the whole mixture until a dough like texture comes (should take a few minutes)

Add some more peanut butter if you want a stickier dough

Form balls using the dough and press down using fork to create a criss cross pattern

Sprinkle salt generously

Serve immediately or allow it to chill for crunchiness

Nutrition:

Calories: 350 Cal Fat: 17 g Carbs: 27 g

Protein: 18 g

130.   A Snowy "Frozen" Salad Bowl

Preparation Time: 75 Minutes

Cooking Time: 0

Servings: 3

Ingredients: ½ a cup of white sugar

2 cups of water

1 can of 20-ounce frozen orange juice concentrate (thawed)

1 can of 20-ounce frozen lemonade concentrated (thawed)

4 bananas, sliced

1 can of crushed pineapple (with juice)

1 pack of strawberries (thawed)

Directions:

Take a bowl and add water and sugar

Dissolve the sugar and add orange juice, bananas, lemonade, crushed pineapples (alongside the juice), strawberries and give it a nice mix

Pour the mixture into a 9x13 inch glass pan and allow it to chill

Once ready to serve, let it sit for about 5 minutes at room temp and cut them out

Nutrition: Calories: 350 Cal

Fats: 0.5 g Carbs: 89 g

Protein: 2.5 g

131.   Age Old Poached Pears

Preparation Time: 3 Minutes

Cooking Time: 17 Minutes

Servings: 4

Ingredients: 3 and a ½ cups of water

3 semi ripe pears (preferably Barlett pears)

3 cups of granulated sugar

Rind of 1 lemon Juice of 1 lemon

1 teaspoon of vanilla extract

2 cinnamon sticks

2 pieces of whole cloves 1 whole star anise

Directions:

Peel your pears and keep them on the side

Take a pot and add vanilla extract, water, lemon juice, sugar, lemon rind, star anise, cinnamon sticks and cloves

Place it over medium heat and keep Cook until the sugar dissolves

Add your peas and lower down the heat to low Allow it to simmer for 15-20 minutes

Once the pears are soft, transfer to a Tupperware with Cook liquid Allow it to cool

Serve and enjoy!

Nutrition:

Calories: 740 Cal Fat: 4 g Carbs: 180 g

Protein: 4 g

132.　A Pineapple "Sherbet" If You Please

Preparation Time: 20 Minutes

Cooking Time: 0

Servings: 4

Ingredients

1 can of 8-ounce pineapple chunks

1/3 cup of orange marmalade

¼ teaspoon of ground ginger

¼ teaspoon of vanilla extract

1 can of 11-ounce orange sections

2 cups of pineapple, lemon or lime sherbet

Directions:

Drain the pineapple, making sure to reserve the juice. Take a medium sized bowl and add pineapple juice, ginger, vanilla and marmalade to the bowl. Add pineapple chunks, drained mandarin oranges as well. Toss well and coat everything

Free them for 15 minutes and allow them to chill

Spoon the sherbet into 4 chilled stemmed sherbet dishes. Top each of them with fruit mixture. Enjoy!

Nutrition: Calories: 267 Cal Fat: 1 g

Carbs: 65 g Protein: 2 g

133.　Very Rough and Tough Fried Apple

Preparation Time: 10 Minutes

Cooking Time: 10 Minute

Servings: 4

Ingredients

½ a cup of vegan butter

½ a cup of white sugar

2 tablespoon of ground cinnamon

4 Granny Smith Apples, peeled, sliced and cored

Directions:

Take a large sized skillet and place it over medium hat

Add the vegan butter and allow it to melt

Stir in cinnamon and sugar into the melted butter

Add the cut up apples and cook them nicely for about 5-8 minutes until they break down

Enjoy!

Nutrition:

Calories: 369 Cal

Fat: 23 g

Carbs: 44 g

Protein: 1 g

134. Mind Blowing Tofu "Mocha" Bars

Preparation Time: 5 Minutes

Cooking Time: 10 Minutes

Servings: 3

Ingredients: 2 tablespoon of safflower oil

12 ounces of silken tofu (make sure to not drain it)

Just a pinch of salt 2 and a 1/3 cups of sugar

1 cup of cocoa powder

1/3 cup of instant coffee powder (decaf)

1 teaspoon of vanilla extract

1 cup of whole wheat flour

Directions:

Pre-heat your oven to 325-degree Fahrenheit. Take an electric mixer and blend tofu until a creamy texture is obtained. Add salt, oil, cocoa, sugar coffee and vanilla and blend it again. Once the sugar has dissolved, remove the mixture from your blender and whisk in flour. Pour the batter into a greased up 9x13 inch baking pan. Bake for about 25-30 minutes until the cake starts to pull away from the sides of the pan. The bar should give you a glossy finish, take them out and allow it to cool. Cut them using a clean (wet) knife and serve!

Nutrition: Calories: 117 Fats: 2g

Carbs: 24g Protein: 2.4g

135. Tapioca Strawberry Mix

Preparation Time: 15 Minutes

Cooking Time: 0

Servings: 4

Ingredients

½ a cup of fresh strawberries, halved and hulled

1 and a ½ cup of water

¼ cup of quick-Cook tapioca

Directions:

Take your blender and add the berries alongside water

Process for a few minutes until a smooth mixture forms

Add the tapioca and allow it to sit for about 10 minutes

Bring the mixture to a boil over medium heat, making sure to keep stirring it from time to time

Pour the mix into serving dishes and enjoy!

Nutrition:

Calories: 51 Cal

Fats: 9 g

Carbs:13 g

Protein:2 g

136. Paper Thin Carrot Crisps

Preparation Time: 50 Minutes

Cooking Time: 10 Minute

Servings: 4

Ingredients:

3 cups of carrots sliced paper thin

2 tablespoon of olive oil

2 teaspoon of ground cumin

½ a teaspoon of smoked paprika

Pinch of salt

Directions:

Pre-heat your oven to 215-degree Fahrenheit

Slice up the carrots into paper thin coin shapes

Add the slices to a bowl and toss well with spices and oil

Mix and lay them out on a baking sheet lined up with parchment paper

Sprinkle salt

Bake for 8-10 minutes and enjoy!

Nutrition:

Calories: 280 Cal

Fat: 0 g

Carbs: 0 g

Protein: 0 g

137. Beautiful Mango and Chia Pudding

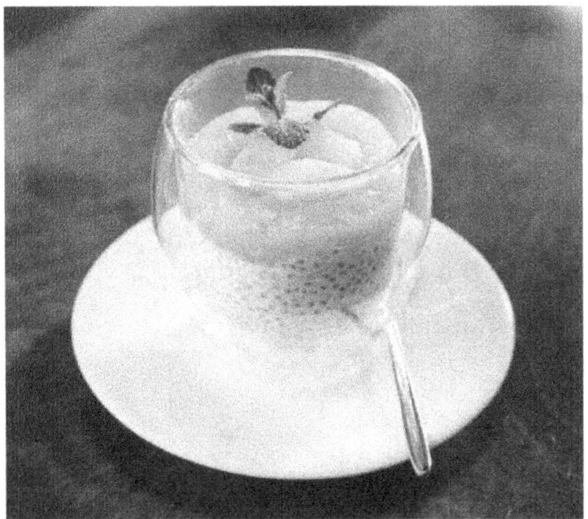

Preparation Time: 10 Minutes

Cooking Time: 60 Minutes

Servings: 4

Ingredients:

1 whole mango completely peeled up and pureed

1 whole cup of coconut milk

3 tablespoon of chia seed

Directions:

Take a bowl and add the listed ingredients

Give it a nice stir and allow them to chill for an hour. Serve!

Nutrition:

Calories: 146 Cal Fat: 26g Carbs: 15 g

Protein: 23 g

138.   Sassy Chocolate Mousse

Preparation Time: 10 Minutes

Cooking Time: 0

Servings: 4

Ingredients:

Coconut cream scraped from the upper side of 2 pieces of 13.5-ounce chilled cans of full fat coconut milk

4 tablespoons of cocoa

3 tablespoons of Agave Nectar

1 teaspoon of vanilla extract

Directions:

Take a large bowl and scoop out the thick coconut cream from the can to the bowl

Add nectar, vanilla extract and cocoa to the bowl

Beat it well using an electric mixer, starting from low and going to medium until a foamy texture appears

Divide the mix evenly amongst ramekins and chill to your desired level of cold

Enjoy!

Nutrition:

Calories: 134 Cal

Fat: 3.8 g

Carbohydrates: 16 g

Protein: 3.8 g

139.   Tender Heirloom Carrots

Preparation Time: 10 Minutes

Cooking Time: 45 Minute

Servings: 3-4

Ingredients: 1 bunch heirloom carrots

1 tablespoon of fresh thyme leaves

½ a tablespoon of coconut oil

1 tablespoon of maple syrup

1/8 cup of fresh squeeze orange juices

1/8 teaspoon of sea salt Salt as needed

Directions:

Pre-heat your oven to 350-degree Fahrenheit

Wash your carrots well and discard any green pieces

Take a small sized mixing bowl and add coconut oil, maple syrup, orange juice and a bit of salt

Pour the mixture over your carrots and spread on a large sized baking sheet

Sprinkle a bit of thyme and roast for 45 minutes

Sprinkle a generous amount of salt and a bit of thyme as garnish. Enjoy!

Nutrition:

Calories: 70 Cal Fat: 3 g Carbs: 11 g

Protein: 1 g

140. Salmon, Spinach & Kale Salad

Preparation Time: 10 Minutes

Cooking Time: 10 Minutes

Servings: 1

Ingredients:

For Salad:

¼ cup fresh orange juice

1 (4-ounce) salmon fillet

1 teaspoon raw honey

1½ cups fresh baby spinach

1 teaspoon coconut oil

1½ cups fresh baby kale

½ of avocado, peeled, pitted and sliced

1 orange, peeled, seeded and sectioned

3 tablespoons pomegranate seeds

For Dressing:

½ tablespoon coconut oil

1 teaspoon raw honey

2½ tablespoons fresh orange juice

Salt, to taste

Directions:

In a bowl, mix together ¼ cup of orange juice and salmon.

Refrigerate, covered for approximately a couple of hours.

Preheat the oven to 400 degrees F. Grease a tiny baking dish.

Coat each side of salmon fillet with honey evenly.

In a smaller frying pan, melt coconut oil on medium heat.

Add salmon fillet and cook for around 1-2 minutes per side.

Transfer the salmon fillet into prepared baking dish and bake for approximately 8-10 minutes.

Meanwhile in a substantial bowl, mix together all salad ingredients.

For dressing inside a microwave safe bowl, add coconut oil and homey and microwave for approximately 20 seconds or till melted.

Add orange juice and salt and beat well.

Pour dressing over salad and toss to coat well.

Top with salmon fillet and serve.

Nutrition:

Calories: 497 Cal Fat: 11 g

Carbs: 24 g Fiber: 12 g

Protein: 34 g

Conclusion

Here are a few tips and suggestions to keep in mind while making important changes to your diet and lifestyle:

•Try new foods and don't be afraid to taste something that's different, unique, or even unusual. Many exotic fruits and vegetables offer distinctive tastes, as well as health benefits that we may not be aware of. Mangos, guava, jackfruit, and seaweed are among some common and delicious options to try. Even some everyday foods that we pass by in the grocery store, such as avocado, aloe, lentils, and other foods that are nutritious and useful can be easily added to our everyday routine.

•Try a new recipe at least once a week, or if you're busy, once every two weeks. It doesn't have to be a complex option to impress guests, but merely a simple 3-4 ingredient dish that you enjoy. It will expand your palette and taste for new meals.

•Stay active and exercise often. Eating well is just one way to combat inflammation. Moving regularly and getting into a routine of exercise is beneficial. Studies indicate a positive impact on weight loss and health improvement from minimal exercise for 30 minutes each session for just three times a week. Walking regularly, cycling, and trying a variety of stretching and strength training exercises can help you develop muscle and tone while improving your health with diet.

•If you suffer from chronic conditions that trigger inflammation, do as much as possible to read and educate yourself on the symptoms, treatments, and what you can do to reduce the effects. Some conditions are difficult to cure, though many of the negative side effects and pain can be greatly reduced by improving diet, exercise, and everyday habits.

•If you smoke or drink excessive alcohol, it's in your best interest to quit both, or at least reduce your drinking significantly while reducing smoking. Since both habits can be difficult to tackle, there are resources available online to curb your cravings, and eating well is one way to improve your body's condition in the meantime.

If you feel discouraged after a while and experience an increase in symptoms associated with inflammation, it's best to check in with your doctor or a specialist to monitor your health and any related condition(s). Continue to eat healthily, and if you "cheat" now and again, just start again. Everyone makes mistakes and changing dietary habits can be challenging for anyone. Sometimes, there are experiences or circumstances in life that cause us to abandon our dietary plans, and this can make returning to this diet, as with any other way of eating, challenging. Always look forward and consider the benefits of following the diet previously, which can be inspiring to begin again.